DEVELOPING ADVANCED SKILLS IN PRACTICE TEACHING

Also by the editors:

Brookes, D. and Smith, A: Non-Medical Prescribing in Healthcare Practice
(Palgrave Macmillan, 2006)

Developing Advanced Skills in Practice Teaching

Anne Smith, University of Reading, UK
Heather McAskill, Robert Gordon University, UK
Kirsten Jack, Manchester Metropolitan University, UK

palgrave
macmillan

First published 2009 by
PALGRAVE MACMILLAN

Palgrave Macmillan in the UK is an imprint of Macmillan Publishers Limited, registered in England, company number 785998, of Houndmills, Basingstoke, Hampshire RG21 6XS.

Palgrave Macmillan in the US is a division of St Martin's Press LLC, 175 Fifth Avenue, New York, NY 10010.

Palgrave Macmillan is the global academic imprint of the above companies and has companies and representatives throughout the world.

Palgrave® and Macmillan® are registered trademarks in the United States, the United Kingdom, Europe and other countries.

ISBN-13: 978–0–230–20558–1
ISBN-10: 0–230–20558–5

This book is printed on paper suitable for recycling and made from fully managed and sustained forest sources. Logging, pulping and manufacturing processes are expected to conform to the environmental regulations of the country of origin.

A catalogue record for this book is available from the British Library.

A catalog record for this book is available from the Library of Congress.

10 9 8 7 6 5 4 3 2 1
18 17 16 15 14 13 12 11 10 09

Printed and bound in China

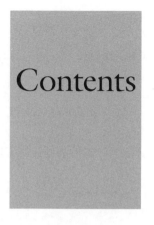

Contents

Part II   Perspectives from Practice

Acknowledgements

The editors would like to extend their thanks to all those who have dedicated their time and energy to contributing to this text.

Anne would particularly like to pay tribute to her co-editors for demonstrating such determination and commitment towards bringing this project to fruition. It has been an interesting journey and we hope that the book proves to be a useful addition to the current literature on the subject of practice teaching.

Finally the idea for this book was conceived by members of the Association of District Nurse Educators driven by their passion for promoting the very specialised role of the Community Practice Teacher in relation to District Nurse education.

Disclaimer

Every effort has been made to ensure compliance with copyright regulations. However, if copyright has been accidentally/inadvertently infringed the editors would like to rectify the issue at the earliest opportunity.

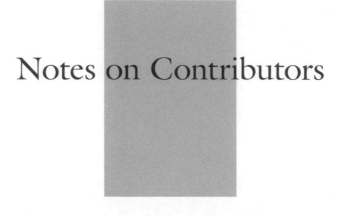

Notes on Contributors

Karen Adams RN, RM, Registered Nurse Prescriber, RHV, RNT, MA, PG Dip Karen is Senior Lecturer in Primary Care and Public Health at the University of Huddersfield. She is also Route Leader for Health Visiting on the MSc Public Health Nursing Practice, Course Leader for Practice Teaching for Health Professionals and Module Leader for Independent and Supplementary Nurse Prescribing.

Sue Boran MSc, RGN, DN, RNT
Sue is Senior Lecturer, Course Director for District Nursing and the Primary Care Scheme Co-ordinator within the Faculty of Health and Social Care at London South Bank University. Sue has worked at the university since 2000, teaching on a range of health and social care courses but predominantly district nursing. Prior to this she worked as a district nurse and practice teacher in London for eight years. She is also a member of the Association of District Nurse Educators.

Sue Chilton BNurs, RN, DN, HV, MSc, PGCE, DNT
Sue is Senior Lecturer at University of Gloucestershire. She is also Staff Nurse for the District Nursing Service for Gloucestershire Primary Care Trust.

Pat Clarke RGN, RM, RHV, BA (Hons)
Pat has worked in the NHS for 20 years as nurse, midwife, health visitor and is currently within professional development. She spent 12 months on secondment at them University of Chester teaching mainly pre-registration nursing students. She has recently completed a Master's Degree in Educational Management. Her research interests include: how mentoring can be used as an education tool to promote and develop interagency working.

Abigail Cooper Dip, BSc (Hons), Post-Experience Teaching Certificate
Abigail is a Clinical Practice Educator for trauma and orthopaedics at the Royal Berkshire and Battle Hospital in Reading. She is involved in mentoring the mentors and training ward staff, particularly participating in induction programmes for new staff.

Carol Fairfield MA, BSc MRCSLT, Reg HPC
Carol is Director of Clinical Education at the University of Reading. Since qualifying she has been in clinical practice specialising in adults with acquired neurological speech and swallowing disorders. Carol was head of adult services until September 2001 when she began a lectureship in clinical practice on the Speech and Language Therapy programmes at the University of Reading. Her current interests are teaching and research in the areas of clinical education, voice and swallowing disorders as well as maintaining a clinical caseload in the University speech and language therapy clinic where student placements are provided.

Marilyn Fitzpatrick MSc, BNurs (Hons) PGDE, RNT, RGN, NDN Certificate
Marilyn is Senior Lecturer in Community Nursing, Course Leader for the MSc/BSc (Hons) in Community Health and Award Leader for District Nursing at Manchester Metropolitan University.

Rebecca Gilbert BSc (Hons) MCSP
Rebecca graduated from University of Northumbria at Newcastle 1999. She moved to Mid-Staffordshire General Hospital 1999–2001 and then to Manchester Royal Infirmary 2001. Her present role is as Senior Specialist Physiotherapist in Vascular and General Rehabilitation. She is currently working towards her MSc Physiotherapy at Manchester Metropolitan University.

Alexis Halloran BSc (Hons) RGN
Alexis is a Community Specialist Practitioner/District Nurse working in Greater Manchester. She has experience in Trauma Orthopaedics, Older Age, Respiratory and all aspects of Community Nursing. Her main interests include Specialist Practice, research utilisation at a clinical level, professional development and managing health and social care.

Sally Hayes RGN, BA (Hons), PG Dip, PG Cert HE, MA
Since qualifying Sally has undertaken various nursing roles eventually moving into the community and specialising as a Practice Nurse. After working as a Lead Nurse in a Primary Care Trust she moved into Higher education and is now Senior Lecturer for Primary Health Care in the Faculty of Health at Leeds Metropolitan University.

Her portfolio is focused particularly around Primary Health Care Provision and includes Health Policy, Leadership and Management and the development of Practice Teachers. She is particularly interested in facilitating the development of practitioners who base their practice on critical reflection.

Kirsten Jack RN, BA (Hons), MSc, PGCE, Lecturer/Practice Educator
Kirsten is Senior Lecturer in Adult Nursing at Manchester Metropolitan University. Her research interests lie in the development of intra- and inter-personal skills in pre-registration nursing practice.

William Jackson RGN, RMN, RNT, MSc, MEd, BSc (Hons)
William is Senior Lecturer for Mental Health at Edge Hill University, Ormskirk, Lancashire. He has had direct involvement in nurse education at pre- and post-registration levels for over ten years. His areas of specific interest include nursing skills development, service user and carer integration into education, psycho-social interventions in mental health and learning disabilities and autistic spectrum disorders.

Paul Jefferies Registered Paramedic (BSc Student)
Paul is Resource Centre Manager and an Emergency Care Practitioner for the Berkshire Division of South Central Ambulance NHS Trust.

Claire Johnson MSc Health Professional Education, Bachelor of Nursing, RN, RHV, DN, Community Practitioner Nurse Prescriber, Lecturer/Practice Educator
   Claire is Senior Lecturer for Primary Care at The University of Huddersfield. She is also Course Leader for the MSc Public Health Nursing Practice. Her background is in health visiting, practice development and higher education. Currently she is involved in facilitating the development of clinical supervision in local PCTs via a skills-based training programmes delivered in the workplace and developing research in this area.

Vicky Kaye NNEB, RGN, DN Cert, BSc (Hons), PG Cert
Vicky is Senior Lecturer in Primary Care and Course Leader for the PgCert Long Term Conditions at The University of Huddersfield.

Heather Knight RGN RMN BA (Hons) PG Dip (Couns)
Heather is Clinical Education Manager for South Central Ambulance Service NHS Trust. She is a nurse who has been involved in developing an education strategy for paramedics in the South Central Health Authority.

Paul Mackreth RGN, BSc (Hons), PG Cert HE
Paul is Senior Lecturer and Course Leader for Specialist Practitioner District Nursing programme at Leeds Metropolitan University. Since qualifying as a Staff Nurse Paul has worked in Oncology and Palliative before undertaking the Specialist Practitioner District Nurse degree programme at Leeds Metropolitan University. This took him to work as a District Nursing Team Leader in an area that crossed geographical and therefore organizational boundaries. This led to a special interest in networking, collaboration and negotiation in case of managing complex care arrangements. Inevitably, managing, leading and being part of a team in this environment also led to further interests in staff development, teaching and learning.

Heather McAskill RGN, Dip DN, BA, PG Cert
Heather is Lecturer, Course leader for Non-medical Prescribing and Joint Course Leader for the BA Public Health Nursing (District Nursing) at The Robert Gordon University, Aberdeen. In 2002 Heather was appointed as a lecturer at The Robert Gordon University to lead the implementation of the Extended Nurse Prescribing course, which led to a secondment opportunity in 2007 to lead the development of a national assessment strategy for all the non-medical prescribing courses in Scotland. In 2004 she also became the joint course leader of the BA Public Health Nursing (District Nursing), which is currently being redeveloped to meet the needs of the changing demographics in Scotland.

Graham R Nimmo MD FRCP (Edin) FFARCSI
Graham is a Consultant Physician in Intensive Care Medicine and Clinical Education. He is also Deputy Director at the Scottish Clinical Simulation Centre.

Stephen Phillips MSc, PGDip, BSc, DPSN (District Nursing), RGN
Steve is Senior Lecturer for Primary Care at The University of Huddersfield. He is also Course Leader for the MSc/BSc (Hons) Community Nursing Practice and Route Leader for BSc (Hons) Professional Studies (Practice Nursing). Steve's background is in District Nursing and Practice teaching with a special focus on leg ulceration, tissue viability, continence promotion and the care of the older person. Steve is an active member of the Association for District Nurse Educators.

Caroline A Ridley SRN, HV, FP Cert, BSc (Hons), PGC Academic Practice
Caroline is Senior Lecturer on the pre-registration nursing programme at Manchester Metropolitan University. She has more than 25 years' diverse clinical and managerial experience in a range of NHS settings. Her research interests include community/public health and sexual health. She is currently undertaking an MA in Academic Practice.

Patricia Rogers
Pat is married with an adorable daughter, Nancy. Post-treatment for cancer (what a difference a couple of years make) she goes to yoga and truly believes it has helped hugely in her recovery from the operation and treatment. Pat swims regularly and last September took up line dancing. Her biggest achievement however is securing a place on the Playtex MoonWalk London 2008, for which she has been in serious training.

Rosemary Shaw BA, RGN, SCM, PT, HV, DN, RNT
Rosemary is Occupational Health Lecturer at The Robert Gordon University, Aberdeen. Her main area of expertise is occupational health nursing and public health. She is currently undertaking a Master's in education.

Ben Shippey MRCP (UK) FRCA
Ben is Consultant in Anaesthesia and Intensive Care Medicine at Queen Margaret Hospital, Dunfermline.

Jo Skinner RN,RM,DNT,PGCEA,MA
Jo is Director of the Centre for Primary Health and Social Care at London Metropolitan University. She has many years of experience in researching and designing professional curricula. Her research interests include e-learning and the design of a prescribing website.

Anne Smith MSc, BSc (Hons) (Dist Nurs), PGCHE, PWT, RN
Anne is Director of Nursing Studies at University of Reading. She is Programme Leader for the Community Practice Teachers' course and the Community District Nursing course. Her research interests include non-medical prescribing, the role of the community matron and clinical decision-making.

Zoe Wilkes BSc, MSc
Zoe is Lecturer in Community Nursing (Pathway Leader for Health Visiting) at The University of Hull. She is the Programme Leader for the new Practice Teacher (P.G. Cert) programme and Module Leader for the final pre-registration core module which is assessed in practice.

Julie M Wright MSc, MCSP, Fellow of HEA
Julie is Principal Lecturer for Placement Learning for the Faculty of Health, Psychology and Social Care at Manchester Metropolitan University. She takes the strategic lead for placement learning for all programmes within the faculty which have practice placements elements. She is currently involved in developing a University-wide strategy to support students with a disability on placement. Her research interests include inter-professional learning on campus and placement, perceptions of inter-professional working, practice-based assessment and online inter-professional clinical educator courses.

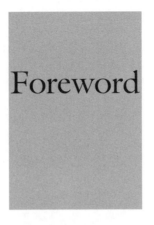

Foreword

The role of educators who are based in clinical practice is undoubtedly a challenging and rewarding one. The development of clinical skills in students, and qualified health care professionals undertaking further education, is an enormous responsibility. Practice educators have to provide careful and expert assessment, effective engagement and negotiation, and clear exposition and leadership in reflective practice in order to assist the student to attain a higher level of practice. More than that, as this book rightly points out, the educator has to be a role model whose own practice, knowledge and skills will be remembered positively by the student for many years.

There is rightly a great deal of focus, both within and outside the professions, on the quality of health care experienced by patients throughout the UK. The environment, funding and delivery of services are always under scrutiny. But the real key to the patient's experience are the healthcare professionals who provide care, facilitate the patient's journey through the system, communicate with the patient and their family and evaluate the outcomes of care. The development, assessment and accreditation of all these skills, used daily in practice by all health professionals, are key to the success of the whole health system. Governments, policies and initiatives come and go: the face-to-face encounter between professional and patient will always be with us and will always be the benchmark against which patients judge the quality of their care. Helping students at all levels of practice to improve their skills in the practical setting is as important to the future of the health services as voting for funding in Parliament or redesigning hospitals.

For the many dedicated practice teachers who take on this challenge, in placements for a wide variety of health professionals in many different settings, this book will provide much practical and timely advice, and a very valuable range of new perspectives. I commend it to educators, teachers and facilitators across the professions.

Rosemary Cook CBE, D Litt (Honoris Causa),
MSc, PGDip (Applied Social Research) RGN,
PN Cert Director, The Queen's Nursing Institute

Principles of Practice Teaching

1

Introduction

Anne Smith

This book is intended to support Practice Teachers in their role of supervising and assessing students in the clinical environment. The focus is primarily, though not exclusively, on the autonomous practitioner working with post-qualifying students but the key principles also apply when working with undergraduate pre-qualifying students.

As this book has been written to encompass practice teaching and learning across professions the terminology changes to reflect the cultural language of the different groups. Hence, in some cases the supervisor is referred to as a Clinical or Practice Educator and the clinical skills development as 'craft knowledge'.

Similarly, the learning environment is described in different terms across settings. The literature refers to the 'practicum' (Schon, 1987) as a 'sheltered' learning environment in which the student is able to operate without feeling threatened or unsafe and this term has been introduced in the chapters that particularly focus on preparing for the student.

Likewise, a variety of terms are introduced to describe the learning agreement or contract that the Practice Teacher and the student negotiate at the start of the placement. This is the tool used to identify the learning needs and establish objectives to be achieved whilst the student is on placement.

The common denominator is that of developing the student to be a proficient professional 'fit for purpose'. This text is specifically focussed on the roles within nursing and the allied health professions although the theoretical concepts associated with practice teaching are applicable across all vocational professions. A medical perspective is included together with a student's view of their facilitation in practice placement. This text is timely in that it relates to the outcomes of the most recent Nursing and Midwifery Standards (2008) for

Stage 3 Practice Teachers. This stage refers to those who facilitate learning with students who are working at a higher level of responsibility requiring higher levels of discrimination and decision-making. Therefore, the role of the Practice Teacher is by implication to explore the student's skills in critical reasoning and assessment followed by their decision-making regarding the differential diagnosis and treatment choices. Within the allied health professions many pre-qualifying students are studying at degree level such as in physiotherapy and speech and language therapy. The educator within the placement environment is therefore charged with assessing the student's ability to analyse and synthesise knowledge according to the standards of their professional body.

Chapter 2 identifies the different professional bodies that are responsible for providing the frameworks and standards for each discipline. If the reader is unsure of these in relation to their own specialisation it provides the references to enable the practitioner to access the resources and refresh their memories prior to moving on to explore the intricacies of the Practice Teacher's role.

This text progresses from examining the personal preparation of the practitioner when undertaking the role of exploring how the team and the setting should be prepared. Chapter 5 is devoted to learning theories which provides the theoretical underpinnings for the educational role of the Practice Teacher and grounds the activities organised by the supervisor to appropriately test the clinical or craft skills of the student. This is followed by Chapter 6 on reflection, the cornerstone of practice development.

One key area that is a common concern for the Practice Teacher is that of assessing the student. This subject has been explored in some depth in Chapters 8 and 9; first, by examining the principles that should be adhered to when performing assessment. Subsequently, different methods of assessment are appraised and their potential considered in respect of the knowledge or skills being focussed upon. Formative and summative assessment is discussed, emphasising the role of constructive feedback.

One particular element of the Practice Teachers' role that instils anxiety is managing the 'challenging' student. This scenario may arise due to the student being over-enthusiastic and too eager to become involved, before they have the appropriately refined skills, or conversely they may not exhibit any interest, never fully engage with the team or fulfil the criteria set for the placement. These situations are difficult for the supervisor to manage effectively and Chapter 10 seeks to tease out some of these issues and suggest techniques that may be useful for supporting practitioners confronted with these dilemmas.

Chapter 13 explores the definition of the 'expert practitioner' and precisely what this means in real terms. How does the practitioner know when they have achieved this level of expertise? This is an interesting debate for those who are leaders in their profession and hold the responsibility for disseminating professional knowledge and skills to those who will ultimately take up that responsibility for following generations. Every student can remember their practice supervisors, particularly those who have impressed them or indeed those who have depressed them with their poor knowledge and skills.

Practical exercises are scattered throughout to provoke reflection and analysis of the concepts introduced in the text and each chapter contains examples drawn from practice to illustrate the points being discussed. There are also further resources highlighted at the end of many chapters to provide opportunities to examine the topics addressed within the chapter.

The contributions that comprise Part 2 of the book have been made by professionals from a variety of backgrounds, indicating the contemporary issues that impact on the facilitation of the educational experience. These offer insights and perspectives that demonstrate the current issues that are relevant to each professional group. One interesting contribution (Perspective 1) is from a patient and this has been included as a narrative that can be used as a resource. It provides the foundation of a case study exercise in which the user or client perspective can be examined.

The aim of this book is to provide a useful, practical tool for the busy practitioners to use, so as to enable them to perform their role effectively. It should encourage the reader to reflect on their skills and evaluate the ways in which their own practice could be advanced as part of continuous professional development.

References

Schon, D.A. (1987) *Educating the Reflective Practitioner.* San Francisco: Jossey-Bass.

Nursing and Midwifery Council (2008) *Standards to Support Learning and Assessment in Practice. NMC Standards for Mentors, Practice Teachers and Teachers.* London: Nursing and Midwifery Council.

2

The Frameworks: Implications for Placement Learning

Julie M Wright

CHAPTER OBJECTIVES

Aim

To guide the reader through the different frameworks and standards that exist for professional practice and for placement learning, and to facilitate the interpretation and implications of these frameworks.

Learning outcomes

- Identify the relevant frameworks and standards for their practice as an educator.
- Evaluate the usefulness of the information to support them in their role.
- Identify common themes in all the frameworks.
- Critically reflect on their own role and on their needs as an educator.

The professional who supports, supervises and assesses learners in the practice/work-based setting is faced with many frameworks and standards for practice and for placement/work-based learning.

Throughout this chapter, the term 'educator' will be adopted as a generic term for the professional who supports, supervises and assesses students.

Why do frameworks and standards or codes of practice exist?

The frameworks and standards have been developed across the health and social care sectors as part of a regulation process to improve professional practice and consequently protect the public. Standards are benchmarks by which performance can be measured. Some are mandatory and some have been set to guide and inform practice. This varies between frameworks and between professions.

The standards and frameworks state what is expected of professionals in their practice. They also aim to ensure that health and social care graduates are fit for award, for practice (e.g. eligible for membership of professional group) and for purpose (e.g. employable to meet the needs of the service and its clients).

Policy context which has informed the frameworks and standards

Historically, higher education quality assurance processes, both internally and externally, tended to focus on campus-based learning. Whilst it is generally accepted that higher education institutions are required to provide quality learning experiences for their students, it is only relatively recently that more focus has been directed at placement learning.

One of the key drivers for this shift came from a report by the National Committee of Inquiry into Higher Education (1997) commonly referred to as the Dearing Report.

Following the recommendations of the report and, in particular, recommendation 24, the Quality Assurance Agency for Higher Education (QAA), as part of their aim to achieve consistency in standards and quality of learning, produced a Code of Practice comprising ten sections. Work based and placement learning has a dedicated section (Section 9), which has undergone revision in 2007 (Quality Assurance Agency for Higher Education, 2007). Whilst this code of practice is primarily for the higher education institutions, it is hoped that the revised code will be used by a wider audience, including employers and the Sector Skills Councils (Quality Assurance Agency for Higher Education, 2006).

Around the same time, there was a drive to modernise health care delivery. For the health sector, the Department of Health publications such as the NHS Plan (Department of Health, 2000c), Meeting the Challenge (Department of Health, 2000b) and Working Together, Learning Together (Department of Health, 2001) have highlighted the importance of quality placement opportunities and the role of the health sector in the education process of student health professionals.

Similarly for the social care sector, Section 62 of the Care Standards Act (2000) placed a duty on the General Social Care Council to develop codes of practice for social care workers and employers. This meant for the first time that the social care sector had similar regulation to doctors, nurses and other allied health professionals.

The Health and Social Care Bill (2007–08), which is going through Parliamentary procedures at the time of this publication, has made recommendations that may have implications for the regulation of health and social care professionals in the future.

Professional, statutory and regulatory bodies

Each profession has a professional body, which represents and provides a voice for its members. It provides a wide range of services which may include support for individuals, guidance for good practice and in some cases, trade union services. Statutory and regulatory bodies have a duty placed upon them by the law (statute) to regulate a particular profession or group of professions; for example, Health Professions Order (2001) placed a duty on the Health Professions Council to provide a register of professionals, to regulate conduct and to set standards for performance for the allied health professions. The statutory and regulatory bodies also set standards for professional training, including placement/work-based learning.

Table 2.1 illustrates the majority of the professional, regulatory and statutory bodies that have frameworks relevant to the educator in practice. The websites provide details of the specific roles of these organisations.

=============== **ACTIVITY 2.1** ===============

All the bodies in Table 2.1 have websites and the frameworks, standards and guidelines can be accessed via these.

▉ Identify which body is relevant to you and the students you support in practice.
▉ Are there any other bodies with frameworks relevant to your profession?

(Remember that some frameworks are generic and some are specific.
Some are mandatory and only applicable for your own particular profession.)

The frameworks should be used to guide practice with particular focus on the role in placement learning. The criteria within the frameworks should be used to examine

=============== **ACTIVITY 2.2** ===============

Evaluate the usefulness of the information provided by these bodies in supporting you in your role.

▉ Does it provide practical examples?
▉ Do you understand the terminology used?
▉ Where else could you find information to assist you in your role as an educator/ mentor in the practice setting?

practice and to identify areas of good practice and areas of practice that can be improved. The frameworks can also be used to map learning, to provide prompts for areas of development and to provide direction to assist in appraisals and performance reviews.

Table 2.1 Professional, statutory and regulatory bodies

Relevant frameworks	
Quality Assurance Agency	www.qaa.ac.uk
Skills for Health	www.skillsforhealth.org.uk
Skills for Care and Development	www.skillsforcareanddevelopment.org.uk
NHS Knowledge and Skills Framework	Accessed via the DH website www.dh.gov.uk
Professional bodies	
Association of Clinical Scientists	www.assclinsci.org
British Association of Art Therapists	www.baat.org
British Association/College of Occupational Therapy	www.cot.co.uk
British Association of Drama Therapists	www.badth.org.uk
British Association of Prosthetists and Orthotists	www.bapo.com
Association of Professional Music Therapists	www.apmt.org
British Dietetic Association	www.bda.uk.com
British Medical Association	www.bma.org.uk
British Orthoptic Society	www.aop.org.uk
British Paramedic Association	www.britishparamedic.org
British Psychological Society	www.bps.org.uk
British Royal Medical Colleges	Accessed via www.medic8.com/ BritishRoyalMedicalColleges.htm
Chartered Society of Physiotherapy	www.csp.org.uk
College of Operating Department Practitioners	www.aodp.org
College of Radiography	www.sor.org
Institute of Biomedical Science	www.ibms.org
Royal College of Nursing	www.rcn.org.uk
Royal College of Speech and Language Therapists	www.rcslt.org
Royal Pharmaceutical Society of Great Britain	www.rpsgb.org.uk
Society of Chiropodists and Podiatrists	www.feetforlife.org
Statutory and regulatory bodies	
Care Council for Wales (social care and social workers in Wales)	www.ccwales.org.uk
General Dental Council (dentists, dental therapists, dental hygienists, dental nurses, dental technicians, clinical dental technicians and orthodontic therapists in the UK)	www.gdc-uk.org
General Medical Council (doctors in the UK)	www.gmc-uk.org
General Optical Council (opticians in the UK)	www.optical.org
General Osteopathic Council (osteopaths in the UK)	www.osteopathy.org.uk
General Social Care Council (social care and social workers in England)	www.gsc.org.uk
Health Professions Council (13 groups of Allied Health Professionals in UK)	www.hpc-uk.org
Northern Ireland Social Care (social care and social workers in Northern Ireland Council)	www.niscc.info
Nursing and Midwifery Council (nurses, midwives and specialist community public health nurses in UK)	www.nmc-uk.org

Commonalities and differences of the frameworks

Skills for Health, which was established in 2002, has a role as the Sector Skills Council for Health across the whole of the United Kingdom. Acting as the Quality Assurance Partnership Group, Skills for Health worked with other regulatory and statutory bodies to carry out a mapping exercise of health care education standards set by a variety of regulators, reviewers and others in health and social care (Skills for Health, 2007). They used the Skills for Health Interim Standards against which other standards could be met. Their findings identified compatibility and therefore similarity between the different bodies in several areas:

- improvement and maintenance of quality;
- resource management and governance;
- teaching and learning;
- student selection, progression and achievement.

They found that most of the standards covered issues regarding:

- diversity;
- equal opportunities;
- safety of patients;
- students;
- involvement of service users.

However, some standards specifically covered these areas whereas some were covered in more strategic terms. Assessment and student support in most cases were similar whereas some standards were less specific than others, for example, those relating to pharmacy education and training from the Royal Pharmaceutical Society of Great Britain (Skills for Health, 2007).

If in general the frameworks are similar, the question to be addressed is why there are differences in practice between professions and even within individual professions. One of the reasons could be that the standards are open to interpretation. This can then influence the overall organisation of placements, the way educators are prepared for their role and the roles and responsibilities of the educators and the way students are assessed in practice.

With the drive for all professionals to work and learn within the inter-professional environment, these differences can create barriers for learning with other professionals (Barr, 2001; Department of Health, 2000b; 2000c).

=========================== **ACTIVITY 2.3** ===========================

- Which professionals do you work with regularly in your own practice?
- Do you think it is important for your students to experience working and learning with these other professionals?

▨ Is inter-professional learning promoted in the frameworks relevant to you?

▨ How can you encourage your student to engage in inter-professional learning?

The following is a summary of five common themes identified in the frameworks for placement learning/education provision. These themes can assist in the reflection on practice.

Theme I.   The training and preparation for role as educator in practice/work-based setting

All the frameworks make reference to the preparation and training for educators in practice settings. Some standards are very specific and mandatory such as in nursing (Nursing and Midwifery Council, 2008) while the majority of others are more general and desirable rather than mandatory.

The Making Practice Based Learning Work project is a three-year FDTL Phase four funded project involving staff from three UK Universities; Ulster, Northumbria and Bournemouth. The first phase of the project, carried out during 2003–04, investigated how educators in practice were prepared for their role. They targeted five health professions, namely physiotherapy, nursing, dietetics, occupational therapy and radiography. They found that whilst all health professionals received some preparation and training this was variable in content, length and academic level. They also identified that learning needs were similar across the five professions (Making Practice Based Learning Work, 2004).

ACTIVITY 2.4

According to the frameworks relevant to your practice,

▨ How should you be prepared for your role as an educator?

▨ Is this the case in reality?

▨ Do you feel prepared for your role? If not, what action could you take to rectify this?

▨ Is there anything in the frameworks that suggests any responsibility for higher education institutions?

Planning and structuring the placement to enable the learning outcomes to be achieved

Theme 2.   Role of the educator

The frameworks allude to the importance of understanding the role of the educator. The extent to which this role is clarified varies between the professions and between the different frameworks. Because of the limited guidance in most of the frameworks, the educator and the student can be left speculating on the role of the educator in practice/work-based learning. The information is not commonly found in the frameworks but may be found in the information provided by the higher education institution for the educators.

========================= **ACTIVITY 2.5** =========================

- Are you clear about your role and responsibilities as an educator?
- Do the relevant frameworks provide sufficient information?
- What other resources are available to you to enable you to get this information?

Theme 3. Providing and supporting an environment for learning

This theme appears commonly throughout the different frameworks, sometimes under the guise of a different theme. As with other themes, the detail is variable between the different frameworks.

The theme can be interpreted in many ways but in simple terms it relates to your role as a facilitator of learning; that is, assisting the students to identify learning needs; providing a range of learning opportunities for the student to achieve their learning needs and to achieve the learning outcomes of the placement; providing developmental feedback to enable the students to achieve the learning outcomes; providing an environment for the students which allows them to develop their skills in a supported way. This will also involve working with colleagues from your own profession and those from other professions to offer the same supportive environment where students feel accepted and respected.

Freeth and Reeves (2004) highlight that many of the benchmark statements focus on collaborative practice. They suggest that to achieve these competencies, the planning and delivery of learning opportunities need to be considered. They give the example of the QAA benchmark statements for social work that focus on collaborative practice. They identify the academic standard 3.2.4, which states: 'act co-operatively with others, liaising and negotiating across differences such as organisational and professional boundaries and differences of identity or language' (Quality Assurance Agency for Higher Education, 2000). Freeth and Reeves then explain how this can influence the planning and delivery by offering the opportunity to observe professionals working co-operatively and to reflect upon the observation. Therefore, by using Freeth and Reeves' recommendation, the statements in the various frameworks can be used by the educator in the planning and delivery of learning experiences.

========================= **ACTIVITY 2.6** =========================

Select a standard or competency that your students must achieve whilst on placement.
- Using this statement, how may this influence the planning and structure of the placement you offer?

Reflect upon your practice at present and how you plan and structure the placement.
- Are you enabling all students to achieve this competency in the most effective way?
- Are there any implications for future placements you offer?

Theme 4.   Assessment

It is evident from the frameworks that most educators have a responsibility to assess the students in the practice/work-based setting against a set of defined criteria or competencies. This assessment is formative (developmental feedback) in all professions but to varying degrees educators are involved in summative assessment. This type of assessment requires the assessor to award an overall mark at the end of the placement.

Sometimes the learning outcomes are not always clear to the educator. If this is the case, the standards and frameworks which relate to professional practice can be used to interpret some of the learning outcomes; for example, QAA benchmark statements for each profession; General Social Care Council codes of practice for social workers; Health Professions Council standards of proficiency for the individual allied health professions and NMC competencies for mentors in nursing and midwifery.

ACTIVITY 2.7

Say for instance that one of the learning outcomes for a student on placement with you, is 'the student communicates effectively with patients, carers and other professionals'.

▣ Identify specific statements from the framework(s) relevant to you, which could assist you in assessing this outcome effectively.

Theme 5.   Evaluation of learning

Whilst the responsibility of monitoring the quality of placement learning lies with the higher education institutions, the frameworks indicate that the educator in practice has a role to play in the process. In particular the focus is on the educator being responsive to feedback and making the necessary changes to ensure effective practice in their education role.

This theme will be explored in more detail in later chapters.

Conclusion

The executive summary of phase one of the 'Making Practice Based Learning Work' project highlights the fact that most professions are dependant on policy documents and recommendations for good practice from regulatory bodies (Making Practice Based Learning Work, 2004).

It is important that the educator can identify which frameworks are relevant to their practice and how they can be used to assist them and their learners. They can be used to assist the educator in providing a supportive and conducive learning environment in the practice setting, which allows the learning outcomes of placements to be achieved.

However, as highlighted in this chapter, some of the standards are too general and the educator should explore further literature on learning in a practice setting. It is also worth noting that a search for literature outside the educator's profession can offer a different perspective. This can in turn stimulate new ideas and identify areas of development, which will enhance the quality of provision.

References

Barr, H. (2001) *Interprofessional Education: Today, Yesterday and Tomorrow.* London: LTSN.

Department of Health (2000b) *Meeting the Challenge: A Strategy for the Allied Health Professions.* London: Department of Health.

Department of Health (2000c) *The NHS Plan: A Plan for Investment, A Plan for Reform.* London: Department of Health.

Department of Health (2001) *Working Together, Learning Together: A Framework for Lifelong Learning for the NHS.* London: Department of Health.

Freeth, D. and Reeves, S. (2004) Learning to Work Together: Using the Presage, Process, Product (3P) Model to Highlight Decisions and Possibilities. *Journal of Interprofessional Care.* 18(1), 43–56.

Making Practice Based Learning Work (2004) *Executive Summary: An Overview of the Nature of the Preparation of Practice Educators in Five Health Care Disciplines.* Northumbria University, Bournemouth University, University of Ulster.

Nursing and Midwifery Council (2008) *Standards to Support Learning and Assessment in Practice NMC Standards for Mentors, Practice Teachers and Teachers.* London: NMC.

Quality Assurance Agency for Higher Education (2000) *Social Policy and Administration and Social Work: Subject Benchmarking Statements.* Gloucester: Quality Assurance Agency for Higher Education.

Quality Assurance Agency for Higher Education (2006) *Summary of Feedback from Round Table Meetings in London on 15 May 2006 and in Birmingham on 17 May 2006.* [online] http://qaa. ac.uk/education/roundtable/notes/CodeSection9.asp (accessed 6 November 2007).

Quality Assurance Agency for Higher Education (2007) *Code of Practice for the Assurance of Academic Quality and Standards in Higher Education. Section 9: work-based and placement learning.* [online] http://www.qaa.ac.uk/academicinfrastructure/codeOfPractice/section9/PlacementLearning.pdf (accessed 6 November 2007).

Skills for Health (2007) *Streamlining Quality Assurance and Enhancement.* [online] http://www.skillsforhealth.org.uk/js/uploaded/Quality%20Assurance/Binder2.pdf (accessed 6 November 2007).

Office of Public Sector Information (2000) *Care Standards Act.* [online] http://www.opsi.gov.uk/acts/acts2000/ukpga_20000014_en_6#pt4-pb4-l1g63 (accessed 6 November 2007).

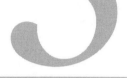

CHAPTER

Personal Preparation

Sue Chilton

CHAPTER OBJECTIVES

Aim

To focus on the importance of preparing to facilitate learning in practice.

Learning outcomes

- Analyse the knowledge, skills and attitude required for the Practice Teacher role.
- Reflect on the value of self-awareness and how it can be developed.
- Explore the strategies which can be used to establish learning relationship

Background preparation

An in-depth reflective self-analysis in terms of the Practice Teacher's personal philosophy, values, experience and educational preparation for the role will form an essential element of background preparation.

Philosophy of care

The importance of encouraging Practice Teachers to consider their own ideology, particularly in the current climate of consumer choice and needs-led approaches to care must be emphasised. Perhaps, it is time to revisit the notion of a 'philosophy of care', which was a very popular concept within nursing circles in the 1970s and 1980s.

Practice Teachers might also like to discuss and formulate agreed-upon ways of working with their team colleagues particularly in relation to the theory that informs the care process and method of work organisation.

========= **ACTIVITY 3.1** =========

Reflect on your own philosophy of care and consider what has informed this? How does it influence the way you practice? Consider ways in which you might develop your overall approach to your practice and how you will communicate this to clients, colleagues and the learner.

Values and beliefs

The Practice Teacher's personal values and beliefs will need to be examined in the context of non-judgemental interactions with patients/clients/colleagues. By acting as a role model, the Practice Teacher will inevitably convey his/her interpersonal ways of communicating to the learner. White and Ewan (2002) stress the importance of Practice Teachers recognising the subtleties of communication which influence the socialisation process. A collegial relationship between learners and Practice Teachers is advocated in which knowledge and experiences can be shared and mutual trust and progressive responsibility developed. They state that Practice Teachers must not simply provide a good example for students to emulate. Students do not passively absorb professional behaviours and values (Bandura, 1977) but need to be active in experiencing, debating and analysing professional behaviour in order to extract personal meaning which can then be incorporated into their own self-image. Clinical teaching sometimes fails to acknowledge those parts of professional competence not included in the technical and cognitive mastery of clinical tasks – the 'hidden' curriculum. Practice Teachers could use role modelling to expose the hidden knowledge underpinning clinical practice (Davies, 1993).

The Practice Teacher should avoid concentrating solely on the technical/clinical aspects of the curriculum and encourage the expression of feelings and reflection on those aspects of experience which complement clinical competence. Practice Teachers need to make the hidden aspects of the curriculum visible by uncovering the cognitive elements of clinical decision-making as well as the intuitive and affective aspects and exploring the potential effects of alternative clinical decisions from all perspectives (Stein, 1984).

Educational preparation

Continuing professional development should be relevant to practice and clearly documented (Health Professions Council, 2006; Nursing and Midwifery Council, 2008). Educational preparation will include formal

mentorship/practice teaching courses and study days which are mandatory in some professions as well as personal reflection and reading/research
undertaken into teaching and learning within the practice setting. An up-
to-date professional portfolio will assist the Practice Teacher in assessing the
relevance and credibility of their achievements and qualifications.

Self-awareness

Goleman (1998) describes self-awareness as one of the five identified social and
emotional competencies that make up Emotional Intelligence. Rungapadiachy
(1999) suggests that becoming self-aware is essential in the caring professions.
Being self-aware is essential if Practice Teachers are to serve their clients effectively and interact well with colleagues and learners. By developing skills of
self-awareness, Practice Teachers can not only differentiate their thoughts and
feelings from those of others but also recognise another person's independence
and autonomy. As a result, they are able to clearly distinguish between their
problems and those of others (Burnard, 1997). Rogers (1967) believes that personal growth involves self-awareness, self-actualisation and increasingly mature
social relationships. Practice Teachers rely on clients, colleagues, educators and
managers providing honest and balanced feedback and incorporate both positive and negative comments. Such learners may also provide a different perspective. The feedback can then be used in re-evaluating our sense of self.

Burnard (1997) describes three key aspects of the concept of self: thoughts,
feelings and behaviour. We are unable to think without feeling in some way
and feelings lead to changes in behaviour, however small. He has devised a
simple model of the self incorporating the *Outer Self* or 'public self', which
includes body and behaviour and the *Inner Self* or 'private self', which includes
thoughts, feelings, senses and intuitions.

Mortiboys (2005, p. 99) describes three ways of applying self-awareness in
a teaching environment. First is awareness 'at any one moment' of feelings
regarding teaching. Second is an 'awareness of your values and attitudes as
a teacher'. The Practice Teacher must be self-aware before attempting to get
to know the learner (Jack and Smith, 2007). Third, there is an awareness of
'teaching behaviours' which are visible to others and could include anything
from communication to habits and mannerisms.

Reflective practice provides a way to develop the sense of self and is discussed
in more detail in Chapter 6. Becoming more aware of thoughts, feelings and
behaviours (Boud *et al.* 1985; Gibbs, 1988; Johns, 1994) can help the Practice
Teacher to become a more effective practitioner (Hoffman, 2001).

The Johari Window is a useful model in portraying self-understanding and
its effect. A four-paned window divides personal awareness into four areas:
open, hidden, blind and unknown. The 'open' quadrant represents things that
are known to self and others. The 'blind' quadrant represents things known
only to others. The 'hidden' quadrant represents things known only to self and
the 'unknown' quadrant represents things known neither to self nor to others.
It is a means of demonstrating degrees of self-awareness. The size of the 'open'

box depends on the degree of insight a person possesses and also how she/he communicates with others (Luft, 1969; Luft and Ingham, 1955).

It is clearly important for the Practice Teachers to develop self-awareness and to recognise their own thoughts and feelings towards their students so that they can select appropriate ways of managing any resulting behaviours, particularly if these thoughts and feelings are somewhat negative or counterproductive.

=========== **ACTIVITY 3.2** ===========

Reflect on your role as a Practice Teacher – include your thoughts, feelings, attitudes, opinions, behaviours, values and beliefs. For example, you could write a piece of reflection or use the Johari Window as a framework and try to complete the four quadrants in relation to your own personal insights or self-awareness.

The learning environment

The Practice Teacher–student relationship is very much a two-way process, and a model based on emotional intelligence is advocated. Emotional intelligence is a concept widely discussed in psychological literature (Bar-On, 2006; Salovey and Mayer, 1990). Salovey and Mayer (1990, p. 189) coined the phrase 'emotional intelligence', describing it as 'a form of social intelligence that involves the ability to monitor ones own and others' feelings and emotions, to discriminate among them and to use this information to guide ones thinking and action'. Emotional intelligence states that to be successful requires the effective awareness, control and management of one's emotions and those of others. This central concept is particularly relevant to the work of people in health and social care settings.

Personal reflections on previous learning experiences, recent research on brain-based learning, Multiple Intelligence Theory (Gardner, 1993, 1999) and Goleman's (1998) five domains of emotional intelligence can potentially provide the Practice Teacher with a range of skills and knowledge within the learning environment that demonstrates understanding, empathy, tolerance and respect for the student by considering their unique abilities (Dwyer, 2002). Dwyer (2002) proposes an educational model that considers developing the emotional, physical and social learning environments in such a way as to ensure that the cognitive benefits for the learner are significant learning experiences.

Emotional learning environment

Dwyer (2002) identifies the importance of ensuring that the learning environment is emotionally safe. Learners may feel vulnerable and, for various reasons, consider the clinical area to be full of stressful factors (Timmins and Kaliszer, 2002). The learner needs to feel relaxed, motivated and valued with no fear of intimidation or rejection. Learning should be challenging and designed in such a way as to allow the learner to participate actively in the process. If the learner experiences a threatening environment, physiological processes within the brain lead to the production of stress hormones. The greater the degree of stress, the greater the depletion of nutrients for learning which reduces the connections between brain cells leading to delayed thinking and reduced learning (Joseph, 1996).

Creating an optimum learning environment is paramount if learning is to be engaging, enjoyable and permanent. The learner should experience 'relaxed alertness' and feel physically and psychologically at ease (Dwyer, 2002). The Practice Teacher should display a caring disposition towards the learner and communicate respect and show interest in the learner's individual and unique characteristics and abilities. Learners value respect and enjoy feeling part of the team (Chan, 2001). In addition, they need to feel a sense of belonging and also to feel valued (Thomas, 2002). In order to promote an environment that fosters 'relaxed alertness', the Practice Teacher needs to consider those ways in which he/she will encourage the discussion of feelings and emotions before engaging in active learning. The opportunity to air personal feelings and any negative emotions or frustrations will help to set the scene for more productive learning.

Cognitive learning environment

Motivation is an essential component of effective long-term learning (Dwyer, 2002). A motivational design model by Keller (1983) includes four key areas of focus which the Practice Teacher would need to consider when developing learning strategies. These are as follows:

- interest – whether the learner's curiosity is aroused and can be sustained

- relevance – whether the learner perceives the instruction to satisfy personal needs or achieve personal goals

- expectancy – the learner's perceived likelihood of success and whether this success is under his/her control

- satisfaction – the learner's intrinsic motivations and his/her reactions to extrinsic rewards

The brain will only retain information that is of interest and links in some way to existing knowledge. If information is to be transmitted to the long-term memory, rich connections need to be made between areas of related information (Sylwester, 1995). When the learner is attempting to grasp a new concept, the Practice Teacher should use strategies to test that the new idea, model or framework accurately reflects the literature or research in question.

Neurotransmitters within the brain regulate attention span in a cyclical manner. High levels of attention are followed by low periods of attention. Hobson (1989) states that, for the majority of people, the optimum levels of attention chemical occur early in the morning and the lowest at night with a low period taking place in the middle of the afternoon. Clearly, in timing interventions relating to learning, the Practice Teacher must take attention levels into consideration. Using a variety of teaching and learning methods will help to vary the interaction between the Practice Teacher and learner and engage the learner. Regular breaks are required (Buzan, 2006) to allow the learner to digest and consider new information gained. It is suggested that these breaks should take place approximately every 20 minutes. Practice Teachers should develop teaching plans that incorporate short sessions where new information is provided, time is allowed for processing and then reinforcing and summarising takes place.

When learning has occurred, information is stored in a number of memory traces situated in different parts of the brain (Dwyer, 2002). The memory trace becomes stronger every time it is used and so rehearsal helps with this process. The Practice Teacher should employ a variety of teaching strategies, such as presentations or group work, to promote the strengthening of these neural pathways. The learner should feel challenged and stimulated during his/her learning experiences. In designing the curriculum for the practical learning experience overall, the Practice Teacher needs to incorporate logical connections between the new ideas and concepts introduced. Learning objectives should be explicit so that learners know what the overall aim is and how they are going to achieve it. A range of methods – discussions, research projects, presentations and peer learning – assist in reinforcing memories. The recall of information relies upon the strength of the memory trace, physical alertness, nutrition and the quality of prior learning (Dwyer, 2002).

Learning is frequently planned, implemented and assessed on the basis of two types of intelligence – linguistic and logical-mathematical. However, in reality, it has been demonstrated that people have a range of different talents. By recognising the diversity of abilities, the Practice Teacher can help the learner to acknowledge his/her talents and strengths. Gardner's (1993) Multiple Intelligence Theory has become established as a classical model in the understanding and teaching of human intelligence, learning styles, personality and behaviour in education and industry. According to Gardner (1993), there are at least seven intelligences or talents. On an individual level, some of these talents are developed more than others but there is always the potential to develop our weaker abilities through lifelong learning. Gardner describes the seven intelligences as linguistic (word smart), logical-mathematical (number smart), spatial (picture smart), body kinaesthetic (body smart), interpersonal (people smart), intrapersonal (self-smart) and music. In his later work (1999), Gardner acknowledges the existence of further possible intelligences which include naturalistic (natural environment), spiritual/existential (religion and ultimate issues) and moral (ethics, humanity, value of life). The Multiple Intelligence Theory reflects a definition of human nature from a cognitive perspective in terms of how we perceive. It also helps in the identification of preferred learning styles as well as behavioural and working styles and a person's natural strengths. Gardner suggests that most of us are strong in three types of intelligence and that these indicate not only a person's abilities but also ways in which they prefer to learn and build on their strengths and weaknesses. People who use their stronger intelligences develop their motivation and are happy and stimulated. For the purposes of assessment of learning, the

Practice Teacher should offer the learner several different ways to communicate their competence and not rely solely on linguistic or logical-mathematical intelligences. By acknowledging that people have different abilities, we accept that everyone is of value and learns in their own unique way. In so doing, the Practice Teacher can promote a vast range of capabilities that have value in life and health, and social care organisations and help learners to grow and fulfil their potential.

Physical learning environment

In considering the physical learning environment, there are many factors that influence learning including nutrition, temperature, sleep and rest (Maslow, 1970). Although some factors may be beyond our control, the Practice Teacher should be aware of those he/she can manage. Ensuring adequate nutrition and water are important as is timetabling learning experiences to take advantage of optimum attention levels and including energisers and physical activities to maintain interest and boost motivation. An appreciation of the richness of the patient learning environment overall will assist the Practice Teacher in exploiting opportunistic learning experiences fully. Such experiences will enhance the student's practical knowledge and skills and compliment more formal learning. In addition, the student will develop a deeper understanding of the value of reflective practice and continuing professional development.

Social learning environment

Managing emotions and making sense of personal feelings is essential in developing therapeutic working and learning interactions between the Practice Teacher and learner. The social environment is a significant factor in effective learning. Goleman (1998) demonstrates that emotional well being is the strongest predictor of academic success and achievement in life. Emotional Intelligence Theory (EQ – Emotional Quotient) reflects two aspects of intelligence: first, understanding yourself, your goals, intentions, responses and behaviour and second, understanding others and their feelings. Emotional intelligence involves managing distressing moods and controlling impulses, remaining hopeful when setbacks occur and demonstrating empathy and appropriate social skills. The Practice Teacher will need to incorporate appropriate learning strategies – such as role play, reflection, case studies and simulations – into the curriculum to enable the learner to make sense of their own emotions and feelings. Dwyer (2002) recognises the importance of creating a sense of belonging and high self-esteem for the learner. Low self-esteem results in low levels of the 'feel good' neurotransmitter serotonin and possibly depression and difficulty in learning (Wurtman, 1988).

An effective learning environment incorporates emotional, physical and social comfort for the learner. Essential qualities of such an environment are the existence of opportunities and challenges, reduced stress, enhanced self-esteem and measures to promote sound physical and emotional health.

Reflect on the environment in which you facilitate learning. Do you consider it to be an effective learning environment? Explore any ideas you may have with regard to developing effective emotional, cognitive, physical and social learning environments for your learners.

Creating a professional learning experience

During the initial introductions between the Practice Teacher and student, it is fundamental in promoting an objective working relationship to adopt a professional manner of communicating. The Practice Teacher should be cognisant of the imbalance of power within the relationship and exercise their legitimate and expert power in a positive manner at all times. French and Raven (1958) proposed the 'relational' view of power in which followers must acknowledge that the leader (Practice Teacher in this case) has access to rewards, sanctions and expertise, for example. The exercise of power is dependent upon the beliefs, perceptions and desires of the followers (students). Types of power bases described by French and Raven (1958) include reward, coercive, referent, legitimate and expert power.

In welcoming the learner, the Practice Teacher will be required to perform a thorough assessment of prior learning and examination of relevant personal characteristics. He/she will need to consider tools that might be useful in eliciting this information sensitively. Professional portfolios might prove useful alongside a one-to-one semi-structured initial interview. An assessment of the learner's characteristics will form an individualised, base-line profile. Nicklin and Kenworthy (2000) provide a useful checklist of areas for possible discussion, which has been adapted below:

- Motivational needs – what works best for the student?
- Achievement expectations – are these realistic?
- Hopes and aspirations – can these be attained?
- Assumed skills – are these confirmed?
- Strengths – can these be maximised?
- Aptitudes – can these be exploited?
- Personality traits – are these significant?
- Physical attributes – do they have any relevance?
- Apprehensions – real or imagined?

Develop a list of questions you may use in a semi-structured interview with your student when you conduct the initial interview. Using this checklist list any information/evidence you may need to gather in support of your assessment.

White and Ewan (2002) highlight the challenges facing the learner within the clinical environment. The student is not only faced with the pressures of the clinical learning tasks but also the complexity of the clinical environment and the demands of interacting appropriately with the Practice Teacher, the wider team and clients. It is the responsibility of the Practice Teacher within this setting to facilitate the learner in applying theory, reconciling the ideal with the real and to channel their readiness to learn into achievable and realistic outcomes as well as to assess attitudinal, practical and intellectual skills.

Learning contract

Establishing an effective professional learning experience may incorporate the negotiation of certain 'ground rules' or expectations of both parties in terms of facilitation, assessment and evaluation. A formal learning contract based upon documentation from relevant organisations will guide the learning process and this will incorporate a student-led approach. The work of Knowles (1980, 1984) and others in relation to andragogy has highlighted the need for some mechanism for learners to build on past experiences and determined needs as they engage in learning experiences. Evidence has shown that adults learn more deeply and permanently on their own initiative rather than being taught (Brockett and Hiemstra, 1991).

Learning experiences designed to improve competence to perform a job or professional role must consider the needs and expectations of organisations, professions and wider society. Learning contracts are a tool for reconciling these external needs and expectations with the needs and aspirations of the learner. Furthermore, by helping to develop the different stages of the contract, the learner develops a sense of ownership and commitment to the contract.

=============================== **ACTIVITY 3.5** ===============================

Reflect on your experience of writing learning contracts with your learners. Consider ways in which a learning contract could provide a supportive mechanism for both Practice Teacher and student alike.

Learning styles

A range of tools are available to assist Practice Teachers in determining the learning styles and personal characteristics of themselves and their students. Although it is extremely useful to identify the preferred styles of learning of both Practice Teacher and student, it is equally important to acknowledge the limitations of the tools used to achieve this if more creative approaches to learning are to be promoted.

In a key piece of research, Entwistle and Ramsden (1983) investigated the ways in which students in higher education approached learning. The study demonstrated that there were three major factors at work. The influences, the first two positive and third negative, are linked to the degree to which learners,

■ are 'task orientated' and have a clear idea of what they need to do to pass assessments in particular

■ are looking for meaning in their studying by interacting actively with what is being learnt

■ rely almost completely on rote learning and approach learning tasks with the intention of reproducing what they are studying.

Clearly, learning styles are highly significant. Three main approaches to learning include deep, strategic and surface. Those students employing a deep approach to study look for meaning in their learning, examine evidence critically, actively relate new information to previous knowledge and are interested in what they are learning for its own sake. Strategic approach means that students see qualifications as their main source of motivation for learning, actively seek information about assessment and are competitive and self-confident. These two approaches are positive and lead to students developing effective learning strategies. Surface approaches, on the other hand, are often ineffective overall resulting in poor understanding and low quality work. With a surface or superficial approach, students rely heavily on rote learning, restrict learning to the defined syllabus, lack confidence and fear failure and are not prepared to look for relationships between ideas (Eastcott and Farmer, 1992). As there are clear benefits for adopting deep and strategic approaches to learning, there is an onus on the Practice Teacher to design tasks to enable the learner to adopt more positive ways of learning if required. Educational literature provides guidance on useful strategies.

In relation to practice education, an assessment of preferred approaches and styles of learning is required for both the learner and Practice Teacher alike. According to Ellis (1985), a learning style relates to the preferred way in which a person perceives, conceptualises, organises and recalls information. Learning styles will be influenced by genetic make-up, previous learning experiences, culture and the society in which we live. Several classification systems have been developed by researchers. One popular tool is that proposed by Honey and Mumford (1986), who have identified four main learning style preferences. They have designed a questionnaire to help an individual determine his/her learning style preference. According to them, the four types are,

Activist: I'll try anything once.

Reflector: I'd like time to think about this.

Theorist: How does this fit with that?

Pragmatist: How can I apply this in practice?

Their research suggests that people oscillate between different approaches to learning from experience. Knowing about different learning style preferences is fundamental to understanding and becoming more efficient at learning from experience. Honey and Mumford advocate the use of reflection on experience as a means to developing a wider range of learning approaches. Gibbs (1988) also suggests that adaptability is preferable and that attempts should be made to adopt the style appropriate to each stage of the experiential learning cycle at the various stages of the learning experience. Tennant (1988) believes that attempts to match teaching styles with learning styles to create a sense of harmony may be counterproductive in terms of educational growth. Some degree of conflict may promote more creative learning by encouraging the student to experiment outside their usual style or method of learning. According to Tennant, the Practice Teacher should employ learning styles theory to help students understand how they learn, to encourage the development of a wider range of personal learning styles and to create a learning environment that respects diversity.

ACTIVITY 3.6

Reflect on your preferred style of learning. Now consider learners you have met in the past. Did your learning style differ from theirs? How did you recognise this? You may now consider including a discussion of learning styles in your initial interview. Think about the issues raised if your learning style is different from that of the learner.

Identifying support

The identification of a range of support mechanisms available to the Practice Teacher at the start of the period of learning is paramount. Such support is not only important during a successful and rewarding learning experience but particularly during more problematic encounters. Support for the Practice Teacher is discussed further in Chapter 12. Support may come, for example, in the form of clinical supervision, peer support, learning sets and links with personnel in relevant organisations, such as a tutor from a higher education institution. Quinn and Hughes (2007), state that although the role of the tutor usually includes teaching and assessment, it can also comprise encouraging and supporting educators in practice.

Conclusion

This chapter has examined ways in which the Practice Teacher can actively prepare for learning experiences with students. Personal ideology, values and beliefs, life and work experiences and prior learning form an essential foundation on which the Practice Teacher can build. Being self-aware, in terms of developing insights into thoughts, feelings and behaviours, is pivotal if the Practice Teacher is to exploit the learning opportunities available in such a way as to develop the learner's potential fully. A professional attitude to learning and the ability to create an optimum environment with regard to the emotional, cognitive, physical and social aspects will help the Practice Teacher to create effective learning experiences.

References

Bandura, A. (1977) *Social Learning Theory*. Englewood Cliffs, NJ: Prentice Hall.

Bar-On, R. (2006) The Bar-on model of emotional-social intelligence (ESI). *Psicothema* 18, S13–25.

Boud, D., Keogh, R. and Walker, D. (1985) Promoting reflection in learning: a model. In Boud, D., Keogh, R. and Walker, D. (eds), *Reflection: Turning Experience into Learning*, pp. 18–40. London: Kogan Page.

Brockett, R.G. and Hiemstra, R. (1991) *Self-direction in Adult Learning: Perspectives on Theory, Research and Practice*. New York: Routledge.

Burnard, P. (1997) *Effective Communication Skills for Health Professionals*, 2nd edn. Cheltenham: Stanley Thornes.

Buzan, T. (2006) *Use Your Head*. London: BBC Active.

Chan, D.S.K. (2001) Combining qualitative and quantitative methods in assessing hospital learning environments. *International Journal of Nursing Studies* 38(4), 447–59.

Davies, E. (1993) Clinical role modelling: uncovering hidden knowledge. *Journal of Advanced Nursing* 18(4), 627–36.

Dwyer, B.M. (2002) Training strategies for the twenty-first century: using recent research on learning to enhance training. *Innovations in Education and Teaching International* 39(4) 265–70.

Eastcott, D. and Farmer, R. (1992) *Planning Teaching for Active Learning. Effective Learning and Teaching in Higher Education Module 3*. CVCP Universities Staff Development and Training Unit.

Ellis, R. (1985) *How to Succeed in Written Work and Study*. London: Collins.

Entwistle, N.J. and Ramsden, P. (1983) *Understanding Student Learning*. London: Croom Helm.

French, J. and Raven, B. (1958) The bases of social power.In Cartwright, D. (ed.), *Studies in Social Power*. Ann Arbor, MI: Institute for Social Research.

Gardner, H. (1993) *Multiple Intelligence: The Theory in Practice*. New York: Basic Books.

Gardner, H. (1999) *Intelligence Reframed. Multiple Intelligence for the 21st Century*. New York: Basic Books.

Gibbs, G. (1988) *Learning by Doing*. London: FEU.

Goleman, D. (1998) *Working with Emotional Intelligence*. New York: Bantam Books.

Health Professions Council (2006) *Your Guide to our Standards for Continuing Professional Development*. London: HPC.

Hobson, J.A. (1989) *Sleep*. New York: W.H. Freeman.

Hoffman, C. (2001) Adding strings to our bow or being here now? *Complementary Therapies in Nursing and Midwifery* 7(4), 177–9.

Honey, P. and Mumford, A. (1986) *Manual of Learning Styles*. Berkshire: Honey and Mumford.

Jack, K. and Smith, A. (2007) Promoting self-awareness in nurses to improve nursing practice. *Nursing Standard* 21(32), 47–52.

Johns, C. (1994) Constructing the BCUD model. In Johns, C. (ed.), *The Burford NDU Model: Caring in Practice*. Cambridge: Blackwell Science.

Joseph, R. (1996) *Neuropsychiatry, Neuropsychology and Clinical Neuroscience*, 2nd edn. Baltimore, MA: Williams and Wilkins.

Keller, J.M. (1983) Motivational design of instruction. In Riegeluth, C.M. (ed.), *Instructional Design Theories and Models: An Overview of their Present Status*, pp. 386–434. Hillside, NJ: Lawrence Erlbaum.

Knowles, M.S. (1980) *The Modern Practice of Adult Education*. Chicago: Follett Publishing Company.

Knowles, M.S. and Associates (1984) *Andragogy in Action*. San Francisco: Jossey-Bass.

Luft, J. (1969) *Of Human Interaction*. Palo Alto CA: National Press.

Luft, J. and Ingham, H. (1955) *The Johari Window, a Graphic Model of Interpersonal Awareness*. Proceedings of the Western Training Laboratory in Group Development, UCLA, Los Angeles.

Maslow, A.H. (1970) *Motivation and Personality*. New York: Harper and Row.

Mortiboys, A. (2005) *Teaching with Emotional Intelligence*. London: Routledge.

Nicklin, J. and Kenworthy, N. (2000) *Teaching and Assessing in Nursing Practice: An Experiential Approach*. London: Bailliere Tindall.

Nursing and Midwifery Council (2008) *The Code: Standards of Conduct, Performance and Ethics for Nurses*. London: NMC.

Quinn, F. and Hughes, S. (2007) *Principles and Practice of Nurse Education*, 5thedn. Cheltenham: Nelson Thornes Publishers.

Rogers, C.R. (1967) *On Becoming a Person*. London: Constable.

Rungapadiachy, D.M. (1999) *Interpersonal Communication and Psychology for Health Care Professionals*. Edinburgh: Elsevier.

Salovey, P. and Mayer, J.D. (1990) Emotional intelligence. *Imagination, Cognition and Personality* 9, 185–211.

Stein, H.F. (1984) The ethnographic mode of teaching clinical behavioural science. In Chrisman, N.J. and Meretzki, T.W. (eds), *Clinically Applied Anthropology*. Boston, MA: Reidel.

Sylwester, R. (1995) *A Celebration of the Neurons: An Educator's Guide to the Brain*. Alexandria, VA: ASCD.

Tennant, M. (1988) *Psychology and Adult Learning*. New York: Routledge.

Thomas, L. (2002) Student retention in higher education: the role of institutional habitus. *Journal of Education Policy* 17(4), 423–32.

Timmins, F. and Kaliszer, M. (2002) Aspects of nurse education programmes that frequently cause stress to nursing students – fact finding sample survey. *Nurse Education Today* 22, 203–11.

White, R. and Ewan, C. (2002) *Clinical Teaching in Nursing*. Cheltenham: Stanley Thornes.

Wurtman, J. (1988) *Managing your Mind and Mood through Food*. New York: Harper and Row.

Team Preparation

4

Caroline A Ridley

CHAPTER OBJECTIVES

Aim

The aim of this chapter is to explore the role of the team in the facilitation of practice-based learning.

Learning outcomes

- Analyse how teams function, and identify what makes a good team.
- Evaluate the factors that influence team performance.
- Identify the impact of team performance on the learning environment and individual's learning.
- Critically reflect on the role of the practice teacher within the team.

Introduction

The widening participation agenda affecting health care programmes has resulted in an increasingly diverse population of learners with varied expectations and capabilities. A 'vortex of permanent upheaval' (Webster, 1998, p. 209) has permeated the National Health Service (NHS) over recent years, and in response to employers' demands for a more educated and reflective workforce. The concept of lifelong learning has triggered an increasing demand for training and retraining.

The charge for, and popularity of, inter-professional learning as a means of preparing the future workforce, challenges teams to rethink current ways of teaching and learning in the practice setting. The concept of the knowledge-able doer (UKCC, 1986) applies to all health care practitioners, and whilst it is important to stress the considerable role academic staff play in supporting learning, it appears to be within clinical settings that some of the most valuable learning occurs (Cope et al. 2000; Pfund *et al.* 2004).

What do the terms team and teamworking mean?

Definitions of the terms team and teamwork are widely debated in academic literature, although commonly they refer to the concepts of collaboration, common aim, designated roles/tasks and issues of loyalty and membership. Teams differ from other type of groups in that members are focused on a joint goal, for example, learner development. The model of the 'work team' (Parker, 2006) is the focus for this chapter, and Mohrman *et al.*'s (1995, p. 40) definition of a team as 'a group of individuals who work together to produce products or deliver services for which they are mutually accountable', will provide useful reference throughout.

ACTIVITY 4.1

Develop a team contract. Aim to create a supportive and productive team environment. The contract should reflect the team's values, beliefs and objectives.

- First, establish and agree ground rules.

- Develop a consensual team contract. This can be in any appropriate format. You may decide to summarise your ideas and create a team philosophy.

- Decide how it will be applied and reviewed, for example, at team meetings, and how any breaches of the agreement should be managed.

Successful teams

Senge (1990) considers the team to be a key learning unit in any organisation, and an understanding of the qualities associated with successful team working seems highly relevant for practitioners engaged with the supervision and training of a future health care workforce. The supernumerary status afforded to many learners has created new challenges for professionals, who are required to explore individual learners' abilities and knowledge, and enable them to become 'increasingly self directed as the educational programme progresses' (UKCC, 1986, p. 55). Health care teams are required to be mindful of Disability Rights Commission (DRC) guidance that calls for communication with higher education institutes regarding adequate planning of work placements for disabled learners (DRC, 2007), and the Quality Assurance Agency (QAA) code of practice for work-based and placement learning (QAA, 2007) refers explicitly to concepts of collaboration, responsibility, flexibility and opportunities to succeed. Nursing and Midwifery Council (NMC, 2008) guidance makes reference to a need for practitioners engaged in supporting learners to 'demonstrate and

Table 4.1 High-performance team

Characteristics of successful teams	Application to practice
A clear goal	It is important for everyone to have a clear understanding of what the learner is trying to achieve and their individual role in the learning process.
A results-driven culture	Celebrating a learner's success can boost team morale, and critically evaluating the shared experiences of teaching and learning will serve to maintain a high-quality placement experience.
Effective team members	Teams need to be suitably trained and motivated to support learners in practice. A balance of skills and attributes across the team will contribute towards successful outcomes for learners.
Unified commitment	Everyone, including the learner, has a role to play in the teaching and learning process. Inclusive environments will engender a positive 'team spirit'.
Collaborative climate	There needs to be a healthy balance between competition and co-operation. There need to be challenges to both learners and educators to achieve more, and quality is at the heart of the learning experience.
Standards of excellence	A team work ethic with high expectations of performance will benefit individuals, organisations and service users.
External support and recognition	Resources, both internal and external, must be in place to support teams to achieve their common goals. Best practice should be rewarded and shared with a wider audience to raise standards for learners.
Principled leadership	Leaders cannot make a team perform well, but transformational styles of leadership are inclusive and energising. Concerned with the 'health' of the group as well as the task, everyone involved in the decision-making feels empowered.

support effective relationships, demonstrate effective communication skills and support learners to integrate into working teams'.

With these demands in mind, it is useful to reflect on the work of Larson and La Fasto (1989) who identified eight common characteristics of high-performance teams (Table 4.1).

The multiple benefits of successful teams extend to organisations, individuals and users of healthcare services. Learning in practice settings is often communal (Price, 2005), and the popular notion that 'two heads are better than one' reflects the idea that many tasks too complex for an individual to accomplish alone, will benefit from the wisdom and collective expertise of a team approach. Successful teams make best use of their excellent communication skills and interpersonal systems, to problem solve and identify better solutions. They remain functional during the inevitable periods of conflict, secure within the safety of mature friendships and bonds. There is open and honest discourse, and a tangible 'atmosphere of adultness' (Knowles *et al.* 2005, p. 120). The challenges from the 'swampy lowlands of practice' (Schon, 1983, p. 43) create many occasions where engagement in the higher levels of Bloom's (1952) taxonomy of learning is required (see Chapter 5). Successful teams enable learners and practitioners to move from examination to transformation through evaluating personal and professional practice, thinking of alternatives and challenging the status quo.

========================= **ACTIVITY 4.2** =========================

Analyse the characteristics of effective/less-effective teams, by reflecting on teams you have worked in. List the reasons for this. Identify ways of improving your team's performance by considering what factors from the lists can be applied to your team? What can you do to reduce the number of factors that may hinder optimum team performance?

A motivated team

Motivation is acknowledged as a key factor in successful learning, and understanding what motivates others will assist practitioners in developing a quality learning environment. The first principle of androgogy states that 'adults need to know why they need to learn something before undertaking to learn it' (Knowles *et al.* 2005, p. 199) and Wlodowski (1985) has suggested that facilitators of learning who develop expertise, empathy, enthusiasm and clarity are likely to be highly motivating.

McClelland (1988) identified a combination of human characteristics associated with three types of motivational need: achievement motivation, authority/power motivation and affiliation motivation. Understanding one's own preferences as well as others', can provide useful guidance for understanding a team's strengths. The 'achievement motivated' individual seeks attainment of realistic but challenging goals, but will benefit from constructive feedback about their performance. The 'authority motivated' individual may relish the challenges of leadership, and will work hard towards increasing their personal standing. The 'affiliation motivated' individual, needs to be liked and seeks friendly relationships and interaction with others. These people make good team players.

Theories of motivation attempt to explain the processes by which human actions are directed, and despite a visible divide in the literature between intrinsic factors (those outcomes arising directly from the task e.g. the satisfaction felt from aiding a patient's recovery) and extrinsic factors (those outcomes externally added to the task e.g. salary), it is suggested that for most adults, learning incorporates an intricate mixture of both (Marquiss and Huston, 2000).

Expectancy Theory (Porter, 1987; Vroom, 1995) considers how expectations affect motivation, and argues that behaviour is determined by the appeal of possible outcomes and expectancies about the future. In environments with an existing developmental culture such as higher education and the NHS, strategies which support self-actualisation and growth are considered to be most useful (Rowley, 1997). Health care teams have a responsibility to provide an environment that encourages and enables learners to fulfil their own unique potential (NMC, 2008; QAA, 2007), and Maslow's (1970) Hierarchy of Needs framework provides useful guidance on issues relevant to practice-based learning. Concerned with people's well being in the workplace, Herzberg's (1959) work has certain parallels with Maslow. His research demonstrated that certain factors, for example, achievement, responsibility and recognition really motivate individuals (motivators), whereas others, for example, pay, working conditions, security and status, tended to lead to dissatisfaction (hygiene factors). He also demonstrated that although 'hygiene' needs are important to people, satisfaction is short-lived, and people are only truly motivated when enabled to reach for and fulfil those 'motivators' that represent a far deeper level of meaning and fulfilment. The challenge for facilitators of learning is to find ways within the practice setting for helping them to meet these 'motivating' needs.

Practicum and quality healthcare learning environments

The experience gained by learners in 'real life' practice settings is crucial to professional development (Cope *et al.* 2000), and changes to the nature and delivery of modern health care services has resulted in an increasing demand for diverse, high-quality practice placement provision for learners on health care programmes.

Schon (1987) described the notion of a practicum and characterised this as 'a setting designed for the task of 'learning a practice'. Whilst the aims and learning objectives in practice settings may be defined and understood by all partner organisations (QAA, 2007), developing a practicum which adds value and widens the learning opportunities for the future workforce, will need to establish its own robust and individualised culture, norms and values (Schon, 1987).

The audit process is designed to recognise and uphold the practicum as central to the educational process of learners in health care professions. Chambers (2006) provokes critical thinking when she considers whether, in an increasingly risk-conscious NHS, an organisations 'performance' is being subjugated to 'conformance'. Certainly, whilst 'placement areas should be audited in line with the requirements of the statutory professional body' (English National Board (ENB)/Department of Health (DoH) 2001), the audit process can, if used creatively, provide a team with an exciting opportunity to work collaboratively and promote its uniqueness and special qualities to the benefit of learners and those who are cared for in practice settings.

So, what are those qualities that support a superior practicum and why is it important? There is no dispute internationally as to the value the clinical practicum plays in the holistic development of health care students (Twentyman *et al.* 2006), and many studies have highlighted the value of effective clinical placements (Chesser-Smythe, 2005; Cope *et al.* 2000; Hutchings *et al.* 2005). The clinical experience of learners undoubtedly influences their ability and desire to enter the workforce as competent autonomous professionals, and central to producing better outcomes for users, staff and organisations are successful teams. Clinical environments support the integration of theory and practice, and whilst professional education should allow for the promotion and integration of knowledge attitudes and skills, such education should allow the learner to transfer knowledge *contextually* in a practicum supported by well-trained and motivated clinical staff.

Commitment to enhancing the learner's experience as well as meeting the needs of society, are explicit in the strategic plan for the Higher Education Funding Council for England (HEFCE, 2007), and the Higher Education Academy (HEA, 2007) makes a pledge to partnership working and refers to the importance of maintaining high standards and enhancing the experiences of learners. Whilst the QAA (2007) acknowledge that it may not be possible for all learners in practice settings to have the same experience, they emphasise the importance of equal opportunity to achieve their learning outcomes, the need for a broad placement experience, and one which is respectful of and responsive to the diverse range of learners. They make reference to the learners' responsibilities, 'to meet the norms and expectations of professional conduct in the particular field of work they are undertaking through their placement learning' (QAA, 2007, p. 10), but simultaneously remind practitioners of their duty to support and guide learners, ensure they are appropriately trained to fulfil their roles and share best practice.

Cope *et al.* (2000) referred to the vulnerability of learners amplified by their novice status. They made reference to the importance of social acceptance to facilitate professional competence, and participants in this study spoke of the importance of feeling 'part of the team'. Hutchings *et al.*'s (2005) study referred again to the value of 'teamwork', and the positive contribution to learning of a relaxed friendly approach to collaborative working. Similarly, learners in Brown *et al.*'s (2005) study referred to the importance of a 'friendly face', and the worth of staff that had high expectations, which were motivating and made them feel 'part of the team'.

The emotional climate of the practicum is hugely important. Non-acceptance prohibits optimum learning (Hyde and Brady, 2002), and Price (2005) described how anxiety might dissuade learners from practising the 'hands on skills that are essential to practice'. A positive attitude towards learners coupled with strategies to make the learner feel welcome is of paramount importance. The practitioner who serves as a good role model has much to offer both the learner and the users of health care services. The substantial influence of personal qualities such as enthusiasm, encouragement, positive facial expression and eye contact, being friendly and actively demonstrating a commitment and interest in the particular health care profession for which the learner is entering cannot be overemphasised.

========================= **ACTIVITY 4.3** =========================

Identify factors that may support learner development in the practice setting.
Work through the questions below. Highlight areas of good practice and areas for further development. There may be other elements you wish to consider and add to the list.

Physical environment

▦ Space – Is there a desk/seating for the learner?

▦ Access – What transport links are there to and from placement? Is it possible for learners to meet their off-duty requirements?

▦ Layout – Is the workplace clean and tidy and welcoming to learners?

Educational environment

▦ 'Learning culture' – Is there support and encouragement for learning in practice?

▦ Welcome pack – Is information up to date? Can existing learners leave appropriate 'tips' for their peers that might support shared learning?

▦ Communication board – Is information relevant and reflective of all learners?

▦ Placement information – Do profiles reflect the culture of the practicum?

▦ IT access – Are systems in place to connect learners to web-based resources?

▦ Access to other areas – Are placements organised to maximise learning?

▦ Learning objectives – How does the team ensure they are aware of the learner's individual learning needs?

▦ Training – Are staff willing and able to engage in opportunities for training that support learners?

Social/emotional environment

▦ Welcome packs – Is learner information up to date?

▦ Pre-placement visits – Are these encouraged and supported by staff?

▦ The team – Is the culture friendly and welcoming?

▦ Peer support – Is there contact between learners in practice?

▦ Timetable – Is there a planned timetable flexible enough to meet learners' needs?

▦ Lunch/breaks – Are these explicit, inclusive and fair?

Stages of team development

'The work of teambuilding is never done' (Adair, 1986, p. 126), and team members need time to get acquainted and become familiar with each other's strengths and weaknesses. It has been suggested that successful team performance relies on the integration of three main areas (Figure 4.1) (Tuckman, 1965).

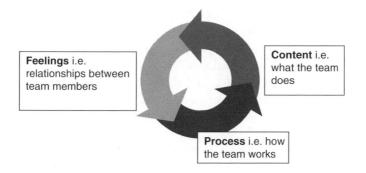

Figure 4.1 The sequential group development model

Adair (1986) similarly suggests that there are three main considerations: task, individual and team. Due regard must be given to each of these elements for the team to function successfully. Progress towards the goal of 'inter-dependence' within the team is undeniably challenging, and in practice-based work teams, a steady influx of learners from a diverse range of clinical professional groups can create a situation where it seems change is the only constant.

Tuckman's (1965) sequential group development model provides a helpful explanation of team development and behaviour. He focuses on the way in which a team addresses a task from the initial formation of the team through to completion, and suggested that a team's capability increases as they move through four stages of development. He later added a fifth phase to address the end of the task period and break up of the team. Within a clinical practicum the model is used here to support the identification of issues for a work team to consider with the arrival of a learner.

Stage 1. Forming – Time is spent getting to know each other. Sometimes described as the 'honeymoon period' (Parker, 2006) as members get acquainted, individual roles and responsibilities are often unclear and there may be high dependence on a leader for guidance and direction. Attention to recognising and acknowledging the disabling effects of anxiety is important in this stage.

Stage 2. Storming – Although there is growing confidence in the team and less reliance on outsider help, 'the honeymoon is over' (Parker, 2006, p. 423). Uncertainties may persist and decision-making can be difficult, as team members vie for position, and forming 'sub groups' or cliques can lead to power struggles. Team members may disengage from the teaching and learning process, yet the team goal of supporting and developing the learner must rise above the distraction of relationship and emotional issues. Negotiation skills are called for. It is important to manage disagreements before they escalate and teams become dysfunctional.

Stage 3. Norming – The storm passes, and this is a time of productivity and fun. Roles and responsibilities are clear and accepted, and whilst major decisions are made by group agreement, less-important decisions may be delegated to others within the team. There is a shared sense of supporting the learner, and conditions for learning are optimised in this stage. Commitment and unity is strong. There is opportunity for managed risk taking and innovation. Ground rules are established and a sense of team pride develops.

Stage 4. Performing – This is the stage when there is attention to 'getting the job done'. A more autonomous team can concentrate on ensuring the learner's individual objectives are met, and the team communicates effectively to facilitate this outcome. Disagreements are effectively resolved within the team who are able to attend to relationship, task and process issues. 'Interdependence' (Table 4.2) may be achieved.

Stage 5. Adjourning – Adjourning involves the disbanding of the group and disengagement of relationships, and is particularly pertinent to clinical work teams who support learners for limited periods of time. If the learner is unsuccessful there may be feelings of insecurity, disappointment and 'mourning', but a successful learner engenders positivity within the work team who celebrate their success and look forward to the next opportunity to engage in the process.

ACTIVITY 4.4

This activity will support you in evaluating the learner's experience within your practicum.

- As a team, prepare an evaluation questionnaire for learners to complete at the end of their placement with you. Remember to invite commentary that relates to all aspects of the learning environment (physical, social/emotional and educational)

- Make time as a team to consider the feedback carefully. Action plan as a team how any constructive feedback might be used to develop the practicum. Identify ways in which positive feedback can be disseminated to stakeholders in order that best practice may be shared and celebrated.

- Can you make any associations between the learner's feedback and Tuckman's (1965) stages of team development? How does this help you make sense of any challenging team issues?

Team roles

Knowing how teams function is complemented by an understanding of the ways in which individual team members' characteristics, strengths and weaknesses contribute to the overall team performance. Belbin (2007, online) has defined a team role as 'a tendency to behave, contribute and interrelate with others in a particular way', and may be distinguished from an individual's functional or work or professional role. Belbin's (1993) model of team roles identified nine distinct roles, each associated with specific behavioural and interpersonal characteristics. Each role is attributed with strengths and 'allowable' weaknesses, and these are summarised with suggestions for transferability to the practicum.

The idealised notion of a team with a balance of all these roles is far from the realities of many clinical work teams that accommodate learners. Newly formed teams may, if time and resources permit, be assembled with all the roles in mind, but existing teams may have little choice but to 'make do'. Caution should be

Table 4.2 Models of team roles (adapted from Belbin, 1993)

Team role	Strengths	Allowable weaknesses	Application to the clinical practicum
Plant	Creative, imaginative and unorthodox.	May ignore practical details and find criticism difficult to cope with.	Will visualise and create an exciting timetable for the learner with new and diverse learning opportunities.
Resource investigator	Enthusiastic and responds well to challenge. Can find people and bring new information to the team.	May lose interest quickly and can be overly optimistic.	Will identify and build relationships with others outside of the immediate practicum, to widen and expand the learning opportunities and placement facility.
Co-ordinator	Confident and positive. Encourages decision-making and guides the team well. Takes on the traditional team leader role.	May be inflexible and authoritative	Brings all the elements of the timetable together to facilitate a holistic learning opportunity. Adopts a calm approach.
Shaper	Needs to succeed. Converts ideas into action. Copes well under pressure. Dynamic.	May be impatient and provocative.	Will challenge the team to improve to ensure the learner achieves their objectives. Will 'fight' to overcome obstacles to optimum learning.
Monitor/evaluator	Strategist. Careful and looks at all the options. A good judge	May be too critical and can seem detached from the team.	Plans ahead for learners in the practicum. Prepares a sensible and relevant experience for all learners.
Team worker	Places the team first. Listens to others. Concerned with positive interaction and avoids friction.	May adopt an uncommitted position during team meetings, and worry too much.	Ensures everyone is involved in the process. Ensures the practicum and learning opportunities are learner centred.
Completer/finisher	Hardworking and conscientious. Delivers on time.	May be over anxious and reluctant to delegate.	Will check the details. Will ensure documentation is accurately completed with no errors or omissions.
Specialist	Dedicated and single-minded. Provides 'hard to find knowledge'.	May fail to see the 'bigger picture'. Their contribution may be limited to their field of expertise.	Will devote time to learners in respect of their particular specialist skills and knowledge. Good role models for professionalism and expertise.
Implementer	Reliable and conservative. Converts ideas into workable solutions.	May be inflexible and slow to respond to new opportunities.	Does not cut corners. Ensures learners receive a well-organised and fitting placement experience.

given to the assumption that even with all the roles in place the team will perform better. Successful teams require individuals who are willing and able to make use of their skills and abilities and this is not always the case. Weak leadership, lack of motivation and organisational infrastructures that disempower staff, are among the factors that serve to block high-performance teams.

Conversely, established teams can encourage each other to develop their secondary role and minimise the negative effects of role duplication or missing roles. An optimistic and positive attitude towards coping with change, both internally and externally, will serve to develop a 'coping culture' that is responsive and supportive of the complex needs of learners and staff.

Conclusion

Users of health care services expect and deserve care from professionals who are trained to the highest standards. Placement learning is integral to the education and development of the future health care workforce, and there is no doubt about the added value and positive influence of a high-performing team working collaboratively with learners in a well-developed practicum.

The social, emotional, physical and educational complexities of placement learning present many challenges to staff engaged with supporting and training others. The task is too important to be left to the few. Everyone engaged with learners on health care programmes has a part to play in shaping the future. When work teams across all settings come together to realise their potential to make a difference, standards of care improve and best practice is achieved.

References

Adair, J. (1986) *Effective Teambuilding.* Aldershot: Gower.

Belbin, M. (1993) *Team Roles at Work.* Oxford: Butterworth Heinemann.

Belbin, M. (2007) *What are Belbin Team Roles?* [Online] http://www.belbin.com/belbin-team-roles.htm (accessed 06 December 2007).

Bloom, B.S. (1952) (ed.) *Taxonomy of Educational Objectives: The Classification of Educational Goals, Handbook 1: The Cognitive Domain.* New York: McKay.

Brown, L., Herd, K., Humphries, G. and Paton, M. (2005) The role of the lecturer in practice placements: what do students think? *Nurse Education in Practice* 5, 84–90.

Chambers, N. (2006) Governance and the work of health service boards. In Walshe, K. and Smith, J. (eds), *Healthcare Management.* Berkshire: Open University Press.

Chesser-Smythe, P.A. (2005) The lived experience of general student nurses on their first clinical placement. *Nurse Education in Practice* 5, 320–27.

Cope, P., Cuthbertson, P. and Stoddart, B. (2000) Situated learning in the practice placement. *Journal of Advanced Nursing* 31(4), 850–6.

Disability Rights Commission (2007) *Maintaining Standards: Promoting Equality. Professional Regulation Within Nursing, Teaching and Social Work and Disabled People's Access to these Professions.* [Online] http://www.maintainingstandards.org/files/Summary%20report_final.pdf. (accessed 21 December 2007).

English National Board for Nursing Midwifery and Health Visiting/Department of Health (2001) *Placements in Focus. Guidance for Education in Practice for Health care Professions.* London: English National Board/Department of Health.

Higher Education Funding Council for England (HEFCE) (2007) *Strategic Plan 2006–2011.* [Online] http://www.hefce.ac.uk/pubs/hefce/2007/07_09/07_09.pdf. (accessed 01 December 2007).

Herzberg, F. (1959) *The Motivation to Work*. New York: Wiley.

Higher Education Academy (2007) *Strategic Plan*. [Online] http://www.heacademy.ac.uk/assets/York/documents/resources/web0288_strategic_plan_2005_2010.pdf. (accessed 01 December 2007).

Hutchings, A., Williamson, G.R. and Humphreys, A. (2005) Supporting learners in clinical practice: capacity issues. *Journal of Clinical Nursing* 14, 945–55.

Hyde, A. and Brady, D. (2002) Staff nurses' perceptions of supernumerary status compared with rostered service for diploma in nursing students. *Journal of Advanced Nursing* 38, 624–32.

Knowles, M.S., HoltonIII, E. and Swanson, R. (2005) *The Adult Learner. The Definitive Classic in Adult Education and Human Resource Development. 6th edn*. London: Elsevier.

Larson, C.E. and. LaFasto, F.M.J. (1989) *Teamwork – What Must Go Right/What Can Go Wrong*. Newbury Park, California: Sage.

Marquiss, B.L. and Huston, C.J. (2000) *Leadership Roles and Management Function in Nursing*. Philadelphia: J.B.Lippincott.

Maslow, A. (1970). *Motivation and Personality. 2nd edn*. New York: Harper and Row.

McClelland, J.L. (1988) Connectionist models and psychological evidence. *Journal of Memory and Language* 27, 107–23.

Mohrman, S.A., Cohen, S.G. and Mohrman, A.M. (1995) *Designing Team-Based Organisations*. San Francisco: Jossey Bass.

Nursing and Midwifery Council (2008) *Standards to Support Learning and Assessment in Practice. NMC Standards for Mentors, Practice Teachers and Teachers*. London: Nursing and Midwifery Council.

Parker, H. (2006) Managing People: The dynamics of teamwork. In Walshe, K. and Smith, J. (eds), *Healthcare Management*. Berkshire: Open University Press.

Pfund, R., Dawson, P., Francis, R. and Rees, B. (2004) Learning how to handle emotionally challenging situations: the context of effective reflection. *Nurse Education in Practice*, 4, 107–13.

Porter, M. (1987), From competitive advantage to corporate strategy. *Harvard Business Review* May/June 1987, 43–59.

Price, B. (2005) Mentoring learners in practice: no 9. tackling learner anxiety. *Nursing Standard* 19(35).

Quality Assurance Agency (2007) *Code of Practice for the Assurance of Academic Quality and Standards in Higher Education. Section 9. Work-based and placement learning*. London: Quality Assurance Agency.

Rowley, J. (1997) Academic leaders: ade or born? Industrial and Commercial Training 29(3), 78–84.

Schon, D. (1983) *The Reflective Practitioner: How Professionals Think In Action*. New York: Basic Books.

Schon, D.A. (1987) *Educating the Reflective Practitioner*. San Francisco: Jossey-Bass.

Senge, P.M. (1990) *The Fifth Discipline. The Art and Practice of the Learning Organization*. London: Random House.

Tuckman, B.W. (1965) Developmental sequence in small groups. *Psychological Bulletin*, 63 (6), 384–99.

Twentyman, M., Eaton, E. and Henderson, A. (2006) *Enhancing Support for Nursing Students in the Clinical Setting*. [Online] http://www.nursingtimes.net/printPage.html?pageid=203298 (accessed 04 December 2007).

United Kingdom Central Council for Nursing, Midwifery and Health Visiting (1986) *Project 2000: A New Preparation for Practice*. London: United Kingdom Central Council.

Vroom, V.H. (1995) *Work and Motivation (classic reprint)* San Francisco: Jossey Bass.

Webster, C. (1998) *National Health Service Reorganisation: Learning from History*. OHE Annual Lecture. In Hunter, D.J. (ed.) (2005) *The National Health Service 1980–2005*. [Online] http://www.blackwell-synergy.com/doi/pdf/10.1111/j.1467–9302.2005.00475.x?cookieSet=1 (accessed 03 January 2008).

Wlodowski, R.J. (1985) *Enhancing Adult Motivation to Learn: A Guide to ImprovingI Instruction and Increasing Learner Achievement*. San Francisco: Jossey-Bass.

Learning Theories and their Application

5

Anne Smith

This chapter will discuss the key learning theories that may influence the approaches used by the Practice Teacher when preparing materials to assist the student's 'learning in practice'. It will not include an in-depth analysis or discussion of the theories themselves. Other texts are available that give a more detailed description (Jarvis and Gibson, 1997; Neary, 2000; Quinn and Hughes, 2007). The purpose of this chapter is to highlight the significance of these theories in underpinning the methods and approaches that may be adopted when working with the student.

This book has been compiled to develop *advanced* skills in mentorship and teaching, assuming that the reader is already operating as a mentor/assessor and wishes to extend their knowledge and expertise in this area. The NMC (2008) has recently published new standards for the support and assessment of students in practice. These are categorised into four levels, stage three being specifically focussed on the standards for Practice Teachers. Other professional groups manage practice learning using varying approaches. In some instances such as physiotherapy, speech and language therapy and social work, health and social care professionals are educated to degree level in their pre-registration training. These factors have an impact on the expectations of Practice Teachers and clinical educators in the workplace.

Who is the learner?

To be effective it is important that learning experiences are organised in recognition of the student's learning needs, the environment in which they occur and the outcomes that are anticipated. Students arrive in the placement with pre-determined clinical outcomes prescribed for their course. It is then the responsibility of the Practice Teacher to provide suitable opportunities for the student to achieve these. It is only possible to prepare appropriately if the Practice Teacher is aware of the student's prior experiences and their preferred learning style (Honey and Mumford, 1986).

Types of knowledge

It is therefore important that those who are responsible for supervising and assessing students have a working knowledge of the theories of learning. First, it is necessary to distinguish the different categories of knowledge. Procedural knowledge is concerned with 'knowing how' to do something, such as learning a new skill. It is usually based on practical facts and procedures. On the other hand propositional knowledge is concerned with 'knowing what'. An example of this type of knowledge is being undertaken here. It is based on the understanding of concepts and principles that guide action (Quinn and Hughes, 2007).

Theories of learning

The theories can be rudimentarily divided in to three broad definitions.

1. Behaviourist theorists such as Pavlov and Skinner acknowledge that behaviour can be learned, that learning relies on stimulus and response. This 'School' incorporates theories about 'conditioning'. However, as Jarvis and Gibson (1997) point out most of the research in this area relates to studies undertaken on animals and hence may not be directly transferable to humans. Bandura (1977) is an exponent of social conditioning and describes 'social learning theory' and 'self efficacy'. His theory is based on the recognition that learning is related to how the individual responds to the environment. He suggests that any learning is therefore influenced by a person's interaction with their social environment. 'Self efficacy' corresponds to the extent that an individual feels they personally can affect this. An illustration

of Bandura's theoretical perspectives can be seen in relation to the topic of health promotion. The focal point is whether the patient/client perceives that they are personally capable of influencing their health and well being. This emerged from Kelly's (1955) exposition of 'personal construct theory' in which he suggested that everyone constructs their own unique image of the world (Perry, 1997).

2. Cognitive theorists recognise that humans use their brains to make decisions and are able to use cognition and understanding to internalise their learning. They also recognise that individuals learn by making patterns in the way they process information. Exponents of cognitive theories such as Ausubel (1978) and Bruner (1960) will be discussed later in the chapter.

3. Humanist theorists expound the view that students should be the central focus of the learning experience, which should be directed according to their needs. Carl Rogers (1969) is the most well-known theorist in this category but others such as Maslow (1970) also belong to this school of thought.

The humanistic approach is probably the most appropriate in practice learning. A student-centred approach will encourage the learner to engage with the placement environment and the team. It cannot be assumed that the learner will necessarily be eager to learn and so anticipating and attending to their needs will be a vital first step in establishing a positive relationship. Maslow's (1970) hierarchy is well known, suggesting at the most basic level that attending to the student's personal needs, the physical environment and valuing them as a person will enable them to settle more quickly in this new context. The stages of the hierarchy are normally represented within a

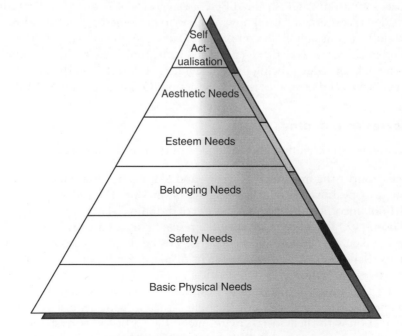

Figure 5.1 Marlow's hierarchy

triangle in which the basic needs form the foundation and the other needs build on them towards self-actualisation at the pinnacle (Figure 5.1).

When examining this model, 'aesthetic' needs are not always included but arguably these must be satisfied to achieve self-actualisation.

================= **ACTIVITY 5.1** =================

Think about the 'basic' needs and the 'safety' needs of the student. How will you address these issues when preparing the learning environment for the student? Then consider the higher order needs and how you will address them. It can be viewed at: http://www.businessballs.com/maslow.htm

The environment

'Practicum' is a term used to describe a supportive learning environment in which the student feels able to try out new ideas or learn new skills in a non-threatening atmosphere. According to Schon (1991) it is a protected environment where students, supported by experienced practitioners, can reflect upon the application of theory to actual practice situations. Rolfe (1996) also discusses how the practicum should be free of pressures and risks, giving the student the opportunity to experiment with some of the messy problems encountered in practice that are difficult to simulate in a skills laboratory. Chapters 3 and 4 on personal and team preparation will have examined some of the attributes of the work area to determine whether it offers an inviting atmosphere for students and whether it has a good reputation for promoting learning.

Using theory to inform action

It is pertinent to consider some of the theories that can guide the varying range of activities that could be prepared for the learner. In the practice situation the student will be exposed to a new setting and possibly a new context for managing care. However, unless they are real novices they will have some previous professional experience and will be looking to see how they can apply it to the new context. This coincides with Kelly's (1955) description of 'personal construct theory' referred to earlier. They will also be striving to learn from the new experiences that may confront them. All this knowledge accumulation and adaptation corresponds with a constructivist and interpretivist approach. The student aims to 'construct' new knowledge and frame it within their personal knowledge base and therefore they are attempting to interpret it in comparison with their prior knowledge. It is imperative that the Practice Teacher does not make assumptions that the student will immediately understand the jargon and acronyms used within the team. This can be very threatening and perhaps one way of overcoming it may be the creation of a 'glossary'. This would be a useful tool to be used as part of the induction process.

============================= **ACTIVITY 5.2** =============================

Working together with colleagues, devise a list of acronyms or terms that specifically relate to your area of practice.
Prepare it as a resource for students who attend on placement.

Ausubel's (1978) 'assimilation theory' suggests that individuals construct or assimilate knowledge according to their previous experiences. Therefore, a student approaching the end of his/her course will already have a wealth of knowledge, although it may not necessarily be in the speciality that this placement offers. It would be expected however, that they would be able to transfer key principles and concepts learned in other areas. For example, they should have some knowledge of infection control. When entering a new area they should be able to identify infection control issues that may be relevant. The depth and detail of that knowledge will vary according to the setting and their previous experience. In turn, they should assimilate new knowledge, particular to the placement that they will then construct and internalise in relation to their previously held knowledge. (Gagne 1985 cited in Quinn and Hughes 2007, p. 84) refers to such a learning situation as, '... when the stimulus situation together with the contents of memory affect the student in such a way that his or her performance changes.... The change in performance is what leads to the conclusion that learning has occurred'.

This also bears some relationship to Bruner's (1960) theory of 'discovery learning' as he recognises that individuals not only acquire new information to increase their knowledge base, but as they 'discover' new meanings they will process and evaluate this in accordance with their previously held knowledge and understanding. As previously described, this is in line with Kelly's 'personal construct theory' that each student will react differently. These theories are of particular interest to Practice Teachers who are striving to develop techniques of teaching that encourage the learner to explore new experiences and to challenge their assumptions. Phil Race (2001) puts this very succinctly and graphically. He recommends that a student who is overprotected but not challenged in the placement will become complacent and bored, whilst a student who is challenged but unsupported will feel threatened. A balance must be struck where the student feels safe to test new knowledge and skills in a supportive environment. This description reflects the objectives of the 'practicum' discussed earlier in the chapter. The assessor will recognise that the student is learning and flourishing as the placement progresses.

The theoretical components of Ausubel's (1978) and Bruner's (1960) work relies on the individual engaging with the task. Ausubel contends that learning occurs along a continuum spanning from rote learning, which is superficial and soon forgotten, through to meaningful learning that is internalised and can be adapted, when required, to other arenas. A particular subject may have been covered in the classroom setting but it is only when the student is able to observe or experience it in practice that they are able to make the connection between the theory and the practice. It is at this point that they are able to 'internalise' the learning. Various conditions affect the process, particularly the student's motivation and readiness to learn. This is implicitly linked to their cognitive skills and their attitude. (Oliver and Endersby, 1994)

Adult learning

Knowles (1990) summed up a great many of these considerations when he theorised about 'the adult learner', as opposed to the child. He adopted the term 'andragogy' which relates to the way adults learn compared with the 'pedagogic' influence of child education. A central tenet of his theory was to acknowledge that adults bring their past knowledge and experience to the learning situation. He also focussed on the fact that adults often approached learning on a 'need to know' basis so the teacher should be aware that the learning should be rationalised and the context provided. Jarvis and Gibson (1997) are critical of Knowles suggesting that his theoretical underpinning may be weak. However, they acknowledge almost grudgingly that his approach has been embraced as effective and meaningful in such professions as nursing and midwifery.

So whilst the humanist theory advocating a student-centred approach seems most appropriate to the one-to-one teaching that is most commonly found in practice teaching, Knowles' explores the factors that should be considered. As his premise is that the learner is an adult, he contends that a climate of mutual respect should be established in which there is joint discussion diagnosing needs and formulating objectives. This recognises that the Practice Teacher values the student's prior experiences and will organise the learning to build on acquired skills. When developing learning contracts this provides the opportunity to explore the learning needs of the student. They are a vehicle for documenting learning outcomes and to determine the action plans for achieving them (Neary, 2000).

When the action plans are being devised this enables the practitioner and the student to discuss the student's preferred learning style (Honey and Mumford, 1986). If a student enjoys observing colleagues and reflecting, then this should be facilitated as she/he may find this a useful way of exploring alternatives or testing prior assumptions. This can be illustrated by a student observing a patient/client consultation and reflecting on how this progressed. She/he may consider how the interview was managed and the type of questioning approach that was used. This may in turn lead to exploration of other types of communication, perhaps the non-verbal cues that were apparent.

ACTIVITY 5.3

Take a student with you to observe an interaction with a client/patient. After the episode discuss how the activity progressed. What sort of communication occurred?
This could then enable you both to reflect on styles of communication.
You could explore non-verbal skills, body language and paralinguistic skills as well as the actual verbal communication.

Whilst some students appear confident and want to be involved in the action others prefer to observe or theorise about activities and make links to the concepts or the evidence base that underpins the actions. An example of this may be a student who attends a case conference and observes the dynamics of the proceedings in relation to multi-disciplinary working, leadership or management theory. The Practice Teacher can then work with the student using reflection and supervision to explore the student's perception of events and offer their own perspective. Other students who prefer to be more involved may like to rehearse a role play of a case conference to bring the situation alive to them.

Domains of learning

Different activities also appeal to different domains of learning. Skills development is associated with the psychomotor domain, knowledge assimilation with the cognitive domain and ethical considerations with the affective domain. It is difficult to separate these as most learning involves all types. They may be influenced by the student's perception of their ability and their 'value' to the team. Initially, they may experience 'conscious incompetence'. Race (2001) describes this as being when a student feels de-skilled in a new area of practice, having previously become confident in a more familiar setting. An example of this may be a midwife who has started a course to train as a health visitor. They may have been confident in their former role but feel very incompetent when faced with their new situation, particularly as there is some overlap between the skills set of these professions and therefore some expectation about their knowledge base. They will need reassurance that this phase will pass as they become familiar with their surroundings and the team.

Models of practice learning

The literature describes a variety of models that can act as a framework for practice learning. It is worthwhile considering how these may inform and improve practice. These models and frameworks can offer structure and guidance when planning placement learning. Students are inspired by Practice Teachers who are good role models (Gagne, 1985). Students are more motivated to learn if they are valued for what skills they contribute whilst being encouraged to develop new skills in a supportive team.

=== **ACTIVITY 5.4** ===

Reflect on how you support students within your team. Do you attend briefing sessions at the HEI about their programme? Do you meet with other practitioners to discuss the learning opportunities you provide? Do you enable the student to work with colleagues to gain more experience? Do you network across professional groups?

Apprenticeship model

Historically, the apprenticeship model was the preferred model adopted when student nurses were in employment rather than having supernumerary student status. It is a well-established model for learning a trade such as with plumbers and electricians. In nursing, the trained nurses were the role model from which the student learned the trade. Rolfe (1996) describes this as the 'pre-technocratic' model of nurse education where the student was part of the workforce and consequently learned skills and knowledge through a 'cookbook' approach. When nursing education was moved into higher education (Project, 2000) more emphasis was placed on the theory and research base of nursing. Students became supernumerary to the team creating a paradigm shift in their status from being relied upon as a member of the workforce to being an observer whose integration into the team was less crucial. As paramedics are currently undergoing a similar change, it will be interesting to examine the relationships and practice infrastructures that are re-organised to support this.

Practice learning is driven by the curriculum and the clinical learning outcomes specified within it. Many professions such as physiotherapy, speech and language therapy and occupational therapy are now graduate entry and this is reflected in the pre-registration training. Nursing continues to have both diploma and degree level entry.

Within any vocational course it is imperative that the student receives adequate exposure to the practical elements of their professional role. It is clear that the Practice Teacher plays a pivotal role in moulding future professionals, in developing their skills and assessing them as fit for practice. This is therefore a very responsible position to be in and a crucial support mechanism to the success of courses at the higher education institution.

Competency-based model

Competence can be difficult to classify or define. Some tasks are observable and their assessment more easily achieved, but some are more invisible or difficult to demonstrate, for example, trans-cultural awareness or ethical decision-making. The preferred model in nursing education is the competency-based model. Students arrive in practice with clinical portfolios stating the learning outcomes to be achieved. The assessor is charged with signing them off as 'competent'. It is vital that assessors are working within an agreed framework to ensure parity. This is a challenge for Practice Teachers.

Another area that can be challenging is the linking of theory to practice. Increasingly it is being highlighted that it is important to operate within an evidence base. Students when in the practice setting may expect the Practice Teacher to be knowledgeable about their curriculum and the theories that they have learned in the classroom. They can be critical about the competence of the Practice Teachers. This can cause friction. The Practice Teacher can find this demanding and can interpret their questioning approach as threatening. Ultimately, one way to manage such situations is for the Practice Teacher to adopt an open approach, acknowledging that they cannot know everything and then using the student as a resource to investigate and report back on the subject.

Structured learning model

Shardlow and Doel (1996) devised a 'structured learning model' that specifically relates to learning in practice. This model is grounded in educational principles and theories and therefore to utilise it to its capacity the Practice Teacher is required to have some understanding of these perspectives. It follows the fundamental principles described earlier with regard to the 'practicum'. The model is premised on four components:

■ Using appropriate theories and principles of learning

■ Curriculum to provide the framework

■ Introducing a variety of teaching methods to facilitate the development of knowledge and skills (based on the development of a learning contract)

■ Appropriate assessment methods that can be cross-referenced to ensure that the student is proficient.

They elaborate on how this can be managed effectively by noting that students' existing strengths should be acknowledged. This model pivots on the Practice Teacher's ability to utilise appropriate educational theories to underpin activities. It is a model that encourages practitioners to be creative in managing learning opportunities. Establishing ground rules can aid students' understanding of how feedback will be given and indicate assessment methods. This will open a dialogue which will encourage discussion of learning needs and negotiation of learning opportunities. For example, the Practice Teacher may consider ways in which to examine the student's understanding of risk assessment in the workplace. It would be pertinent to discuss this with the student and negotiate the approach that may be used. The student could explore the area and read local policies. If more advanced in their training they could then be asked about how risk assessment should be managed and monitored. The Practice Teacher should adopt approaches that appropriately assess the topic from a variety of perspectives, rather than rely on one method of assessment, in order to gain a holistic view of the student's ability. This learning and assessment should be non-threatening so that the student feels able to identify and analyse issues in a creative way without fear of being criticised.

Experiential learning and models of reflection and assessment

Experiential learning is a key technique adopted by Practice Teachers. It is also vital to consider how students learn, indeed they often require guidance on learning to learn (Jarvis and Gibson, 1997). Linked to this is their perception of themselves, their self-awareness and self-concept (Jack and Smith, 2007). Kolb's experiential learning cycle is well known as a tool for encouraging reflection on experience followed by an examination of the relevant theory or research base that impact on it. This in turn leads to a consideration of whether the same approach would be used on a future occasion or whether practice can be changed and improved.

Often in the community setting practitioners are isolated and confronted with dilemmas associated with lack of suitable equipment to carry out tasks and with no resources readily available. In these circumstances they are required to 'reflect in action' (Schon, 1991) and (as Kolb terms the final part of the cycle) 'actively experiment'. The Practice Teacher can be defined as a coach, or a catalyst, and so on, and is charged with the task of making learning memorable and meaningful. Ultimately, the student is assessed with regard to achieving a level of competence but the reward is to be found when, as a Practice Teacher, you recognise that the student has progressed beyond that and has accomplished a 'perspective transformation' as described by Mezirow (1981). It refers to an awakening to the realisation of the wider agenda that is concerned with the questioning of stereotypes, assumptions and value systems.

Taxonomies of achievement

The learning theories have been considered and some practice models explored. However, this chapter would not be complete without highlighting the more widely used taxonomies that guide the process and assessment of learning. The term 'taxonomy' refers to a classification system or framework. Bloom's taxonomy of cognition has some roots in behavioural theory and was originally intended to be a generic framework for setting educational objectives, but later other authors devised taxonomies relating more specifically to achievement in the psychomotor (Harrow, 1972) and affective (Krathwohl *et al.* 1964) domains. Bloom's taxonomy gives clear descriptors by which to assess students' comprehension, analysis and synthesis of knowledge. Key criteria are covered along a continuum within each taxonomy.

Bloom's taxonomy provides a useful guide to the development of cognitive skills starting with acquisition of knowledge at the most basic level (Table 5.1).

A further taxonomy described by Gagne relates to a hierarchy of eight 'types' of learning, the pinnacle of which concerns higher order skills such as problem solving. According to Mezirow (1981) it is the demonstration of critical awareness and decision-making skills that define the autonomous professional practitioner.

Steinaker and Bell (1979) devised an experiential taxonomy that has previously been adopted as a framework for assessment of students in clinical practice. It indicates both the role of the supervisor and the student. It clearly acknowledges that as the student grows in confidence they in turn may become the facilitator of learning for more junior peers. The taxonomy commences with 'exposure' to the setting or the learning activity. It moves through various stages where the learner becomes increasingly competent to the point where she/he is able to disseminate or facilitate learning. This taxonomy offers plenty of scope. Whilst it would not be expected that every student should become so competent and confident that they can take responsibility for dissemination

Table 5.1 Bloom's taxonomy

Level	Criteria	Cognitive Skills
Level 1	Knowledge	The student may only be able to regurgitate the facts and not be aware of their significance.
Level 2	Comprehension	The student may show greater understanding by demonstrating how the knowledge can be interpreted or how it connects with other knowledge.
Level 3	Application	The student will be able to articulate how knowledge can be applied to certain circumstances or in certain situations.
Level 4	Analysis	The student will be able to analyse the benefits or negative aspects of the situation and make comparisons with other possible solutions.
Level 5	Synthesis	The student who has achieved this level of cognition is able to visualise how this knowledge integrates with other previously held knowledge or can conceptualise how this will build into a framework to aid more complex decision-making.
Level 6	Evaluation	This is the final category in Bloom's taxonomy where the student demonstrates that they are able to critically reflect on how this knowledge has enhanced their practice or otherwise.

of knowledge or skills, it has the potential to identify those students who will emerge as leaders within the profession and affords opportunities to nurture and develop such potential.

Conclusion

This chapter has touched on educational theories and models of learning that comprise the essential foundation stones of any programme of learning. In the practice environment the Practice Teacher is charged with the responsibility of providing a secure 'practicum' where the student can be supported to test hypotheses and be enabled to develop competence. There is always an element of risk if challenging the student but, if managed effectively, this translates into providing a stimulating experience. The crucial point is to know where the boundary lies and when the limit has been reached which only comes with experience. This book is concerned with developing 'advanced skills' in practice teaching which means getting out of the 'comfort zone' associated with ritual and routine methods of teaching and facilitation. Instead it is an invitation to experiment with new ways of engaging and teaching the student.

This chapter clearly identifies the critical role played by the Practice Teacher. It is not something that can be taken on without adequate preparation or regular updating. The Practice Teacher is one part of a tri-partite relationship. It is important to forge and foster links with clinical link tutors or personal tutors of students. Different professional groups manage this in different ways but for the benefit of the student's welfare and progression this communication channel should be maintained.

Further reading

A web site is available with various resources such as lesson plan templates at http://www. nelsonthornes.com/nursing/ppne/lesson_planning.htm

This book has a useful chapter on writing–learning contracts

Chapter 2 Strategy for Learning

Neary, M. (2000) *Teaching, Assessing and Evaluation for Clinical Competence. A Practical Guide for Practitioners and Teachers.* Cheltenham: Nelson Thornes.

References

Ausubel, D. (1978) *Educational Psychology: A Cognitive View.* New York: Rinehart and Winston.

Bandura, A. (1977) *Social Learning Theory.* Englewood Cliffs NJ: Prentice Hall.

Bloom, B. (1956) *Taxonomy of Educational Objectives.* New York: Longman.

Bruner, J. (1960) *The Process of Education.* Cambridge MA: Harvard University Press.

Gagne, R. (1985) *The Conditions of Learning and Theory of Instruction.* New York. Holt Rinehart and Winston (2007) in Quinn, F. and Hughes, S. (2007) *Quinn's Principles and Practice of Nurse Education.* 5th edn. Cheltenham: Nelson Thornes.

Harrow, A. (1972) *A Taxonomy of the Psychomotor Domain.* New York: Mackay.

Honey, P. and Mumford, A. (1986) *Manual of Learning Styles.* Berkshire: Honey and Mumford.

Jack, K. and Smith, A. (2007) Promoting self-awareness in nursing practice. *Nursing Standard.* 21(32), 47–52.

Jarvis, P. and Gibson, S. (1997) *The Teacher Practitioner and Mentor.* 2nd edn. Cheltenham: Nelson Thornes.

Kelly, G. (1955) *The Psychology of Personal Constructs.* New York: Norton.

Knowles, M. (1990) *The Adult Learner. A Neglected Species* 4th edn. Houston: Gulf Pub.

Kolb, D. (1984) *Experiential Learning. Experience as a Source of Learning and Development.* Englewood Cliffs NJ: Prentice Hall.

Krathwohl, D., Bloom, B. and Masia, B. (1964) *A Taxonomy of Educational Objectives: The Classification of Educational Goals Handbook 2 Affective Domain* New York: Mackay.

Maslow, A. (1970) *Motivation and Personality.* New York: Harper and Row.

Mezirow J. (1981) A critical theory of adult learning and education. *Adult Education.* 32 (1), 3–24. http://216.239.59.104/search?q=cache:5E5ul_4Too4J:www.ed.psu.edu/CI/Journals/1998AETS/s2_1_dibiase.rtf+mezirow+perspective+transformation&hl=en&ct=clnk&cd=2&gl=uk (accessed 28 May 2008).

Neary, M. (2000) *Teaching, Assessing and Evaluation for Clinical Competence. A Practical Guide for Practitioners and Teachers.* Cheltenham: Nelson Thornes.

Nursing and Midwifery Council (2006) *Standards to Support Learning and Assessment in Practice: NMC Standards for Mentors, Practice Teachers and Teachers.* London: NMC.

Oliver, R. and Endersby, C. (1994) *Teaching and Assessing Nurses. A Handbook for Preceptors.* London: Bailliere Tindall.

Pavlov I. (1927) *Conditioned Reflexes.* Oxford: OUP.

Perry, A. (ed.) (1997) *Nursing. A Knowledge Base for Practice.* 2nd edn. London: Arnold.

Quinn, F. and Hughes, S. (2007) *Quinn's Principles and Practice of Nurse Education.* 5th edn. Cheltenham: Nelson Thornes.

Race, P. (2001) *Never Mind the Teaching Feel the Learning.* SEDA.

Rogers, C. (1969) *Freedom to Learn*. Ohio IL: Merrill.

Rolfe, G. (1996) *Closing the Theory – Practice Gap. A New Paradigm for Nursing*. Oxford: Butterworth Heinemann.

Schon, D. (1991) *The Reflective Practitioner: How Professionals Think in Action* 2nd edn. London: Temple Smith.

Shardlow, S. and Doel, M. (1996) *Practice Learning and Teaching*. Basingstoke: MacMillan Press.

Skinner B. (1971) *Beyond Freedom and Dignity*. New York: Alfred Knopf.

Steinaker, N. and Bell, M. (1979) *The Experiential Taxonomy: A New Approach to Teaching and Learning*. New York: Academic Press.

Reflective Practice and Portfolio Development

Anne Smith and Kirsten Jack

CHAPTER OBJECTIVES

Aim

The aim of this chapter is to consider how reflection can enable the individual to explore their practice within practice teaching.

Learning outcomes

- Explore definitions of reflection.
- Critically appraise reflection as a method of evidencing practice.
- Discuss how portfolios may be developed to demonstrate competence.
- Examine the use of portfolios across health and social care professions.
- Evaluate the pragmatic aspects of compiling a portfolio.

Introduction

The aim of this chapter is to consider how reflection can enable the individual to explore their practice. It will not focus on how 'to do' reflection. It is the intention to discuss how reflection can provide the Practice Teacher with the opportunity to examine their own practice and how to use reflective techniques to encourage critical dialogue with the student. Jarvis (1992, p. 174) stated that 'reflective practice is more than thoughtful practice. It is a form of practice that seeks to problematise many situations of professional performance so that they become potential learning situations'. This highlights how a practice environment can promote learning for the student through the structuring of learning opportunities. It is important to remember that reflection can be utilised to examine both positive and negative experiences as it is so often only initiated following an 'incident' or negative experience. It can be a useful assessment tool, although difficulties may be encountered.

This chapter will move on to discuss how the compilation of portfolios can be used to provide evidence of the development of skills and competence and demonstrate learning. In many of the vocational professions this has become an accepted method of assessment but again it can become a paper exercise that fails to fully demonstrate competence. Across health and social care professions there is a requirement to keep a portfolio of evidence of ongoing professional updating and development to continue with registration (HPC, 2006; NMC, 2008).

The use of reflection as a way of demonstrating competence has gained popularity within the Health and Social Care professions in the last decade. It is increasingly being adopted across the caring professions as a method of demonstrating the critical contribution of experiential learning within the curriculum to enable students to qualify 'fit for purpose' (DOH, 1999; Thompson, 2006).

ACTIVITY 6.1

Consider how you currently explore your practice. Do you use reflection to facilitate this exploration? How do you record your thoughts and feelings? It may be that you don't write this down. Think of a recent incident that caused you to stop and consider your thoughts, feelings or actions. Write an account of it, providing as much detail as you can.

Reflective practice has become a familiar activity within the nursing curriculum for some time (Pearce, 2003). Doel and Shardlow (2005) report the shift in the emphasis of Social Work education in the past decade. Formerly focussed on training to achieve six core competencies, the curriculum has moved to a more eclectic approach, centred on adult learning theory, related to placing the learning within the context in which it occurred. It concentrates on the broader picture as opposed to training for functionality. Reflection has been used as a vehicle to demonstrate this.

It is therefore clear that reflective practice has been influential on the development of professional education (Clegg *et al.* 2002). Some authors show concern about the lack of evidence to support its use (Burnard, 2005; Paget, 2001) and question its effect on learning and patient care (Moon, 2000). However, as stated by Rolfe (2002) if reflection is going to be measured in terms of its technical rationality then quite clearly it will not be highly valued. Reflective practice needs to be acknowledged for what it is, not what it is not, and not be viewed as the poor relation to the more dominant positivist paradigm. Indeed, qualitative studies have shown that reflective thinking is useful to practice (Smith and Jack, 2005; Teekman, 2000) and journal writing can be useful to promote reflective thinking and learning (Chimera, 2006).

What is reflection?

Jarvis (1992, p. 147) considers that 'reflective practice' is 'a frequently used but infrequently defined concept'. Therefore it is the intention here to present several definitions from the literature for the reader to consider.

Boud *et al.* (1985, p. 18) describe reflection as 'a form of response of the learner to experience...after the experience there occurs a processing phase: this is the area of reflection'. It is the link between the two that is important if learning is to occur and time can be set aside to facilitate this process.

Atkins and Murphy (1994, p. 50) also highlight the deliberate nature of reflection by stating that it is 'a complex and deliberate process of thinking about and interpreting experience in order to learn from it. This is a conscious process which does not occur automatically, but is in response to experience and with a definite purpose.'

Boyd and Fayles (1983) cited in Powell (1989), define it as a process whereby the individual internally examines an issue of concern that has been triggered by an experience, which results in a changed conceptual perspective. Emphasis here is on the change in personal perspective which occurs as a result of the process. This could be a change in thinking or the way one views a situation for example. However, it is not only issues of concern which should initiate reflection. Positive aspects of practice could be reviewed, although practitioners may not necessarily value and therefore reflect on situations which went well (Tripp, 1993).

The concept of reflection has been described in the literature for many years dating back to work by Dewey in 1933, but became more prominent within nursing in the early 1990s. Of particular importance is the work of Schon (1987) who challenged the dominance of technical rationality arguing that many of the problems that professionals encounter are not clear cut and are not easy to solve using scientific method. Professionals very often deal in the 'swampy lowlands' of practice which are unique messy situations and require the professional to use experience, intuition and feeling to help them decide on a course of action. Reflection can take place in or on action, reflecting in action being seen as the more challenging. Reflection in action requires the individual to adjust their practice whilst it is taking place which requires a certain amount of skill and self-awareness. Reflection on action occurs after the event has taken place when the professional explores their actions, thoughts and feelings and learns from them. Of course, when looking back at an event it may be easy to view it through rose coloured glasses or in a much more negative way. Anxiety can influence memory of a situation (Newell, 1992) and hindsight bias could restrict learning from reflection (Jones, 1995). Reflection on action may involve challenging deeply held beliefs and values. This may be upsetting as the professional challenges certain actions taken in a situation but unless practice is challenged and confronted, learning may not take place (Argyris, 1994). The potential for harm however should not be trivialised and the risks the professional takes when reflecting on potentially painful aspects of practice should be acknowledged. Facilitators need to be able to support individuals who are dealing with potentially uncomfortable issues (Haddock, 1997). Thompson (2006) concludes that reflection is a 'messy activity'. He refers to the fact that it is not based on the use of pre-organised lesson plans or the like but involves the management of situations that may be difficult to control and also involve risk. This can prove challenging especially for the novice teacher.

================== **ACTIVITY 6.2** ==================

Evaluate the account that you wrote for the previous activity and think about whether it did involve some of the issues highlighted here such as making you feel uncomfortable or alternatively providing a clear action plan for the future. Was the account describing something positive or negative? Did it demonstrate your knowledge and skills or highlight a deficit that could be addressed?

Reflection through journal writing, can initiate an exploration of feelings and working practice that can aid personal growth, and has been used to facilitate development of self-awareness (Chimera, 2006). Ultimately it can encourage the practitioner to work in new and more creative ways. Perhaps one particular advantage of the process is that individuals stop and think about the routine and the ritual practice. It is imperative for all professionals to examine the evidence and their own experiential base from which they operate, to recognise their accountability and to practice in a safe and effective way. Reflection 'on practice' or even 'in practice' (Schon, 1983) therefore is a potent device to accomplish this. Nurses comment that they routinely reflect informally on their practice, for example, in the car on the way home (Smith and Jack, 2005). This may not necessarily lead to constructive analysis and action or a change in practice. However, it may provide a method of problem solving for the practitioner after a busy day. Boud *et al.* (1985) also suggest that although personal reflection can be helpful, reflection that is facilitated by a good listener with appropriate technical skills will engender a more in-depth examination. This may enable the student to consider alternative interpretations of their perceptions, consciously examine their non-verbal behaviours or seek information concerning the situation under discussion. Skilled facilitation is not easy to perform (Heron, 1990). The Practice Teacher must also be sensitive to her own personal presentation and behaviour.

Models of reflection

From an academic perspective students may be advised to reflect using a structured model to organise their thoughts and formulate their future plans. This can constrain creative thought making the whole process an academic exercise and not truly fulfilling the function for which it was initiated (Hargreaves, 2004; Scholes *et al.* 2004). Therefore it is pertinent to consider some of the models described in the literature. This will enable the Practice Teacher to determine whether the use of a model of reflection could assist them in their role.

Boud *et al.* (1985) pointed out that subconscious reflection is a regular occurrence but it is only when it is formalised that it becomes a learning experience. Thus, models of reflection such as Gibbs (1988) and Kolb (1984) are taught as frameworks to initiate a more structured approach.

Taylor's model (1987) was adopted and adapted by Dewar and Walker (1999) and recognises the emotional constituent of reflection in which the student may become disorientated, which can be a threatening experience. The importance of the use of emotion in health care practice cannot be underestimated (Freshwater and Stickley, 2004) The Practice Teacher must be sensitive to the student's reaction in such circumstances.

Faugier's 'growth and support model (1994) is based on the humanistic philosophy that prioritises the student's development. It is a 'process model' that considers how the student should be supported to develop holistically, rather than a tick-list approach to accomplish the competencies. Boud *et al.* (1985) make reference to the fact that experience should not be a passive observation but an active engagement for the student.

Mezirow (1981) suggests seven levels of reflection starting with reflectivity, which is being aware of and being able to describe experiences. The seventh level is more critical and theoretical when one is not only aware of experiences, but is able to challenge the influence of assumptions on experiences in practice. Coutts-Jarman (1993) suggested five categories of reflectivity commencing with awareness of how experiences affect the individual on a personal level through a taxonomy to a very analytical stance that she termed 'psychic reflectivity'. At this level the individual is able to critically acknowledge the limitations that may impact on the activity. These may be due to selection, manipulation or other forces that determine how an event may be conceptualised and interpreted. This is a good observation as it may be that the novice learner has a restricted comprehension due to lack of professional knowledge when analysing practice. In contrast, the expert practitioner has the ability to act intuitively (Benner and Tanner 1987 cited in Palmer *et al.* 1994) because they have developed such expert knowledge to inform their actions that they operate almost automatically. The student when observing the 'expert practitioner' cannot always perceive how the decisions have been made as the practitioner is not transparently exhibiting the decision-making process, leaving the student perplexed. The Practice Teacher will need to be aware that when working with the student their decision-making trail may require explaining in order to use such instances as a learning experience for the student. This concept is graphically encapsulated by Benner (1984) who wrote of the journey from 'novice' to 'expert'.

Thus, reflection is a vehicle for analysing the experiential knowledge that informs practice. It can be used as a tool by the Practice Teacher during the process of supervision and assessment of the student. This chapter will now examine how reflection can contribute to the evidence that is generated when developing a portfolio.

═══════════════════════ **ACTIVITY 6.3** ═══════════════════════

Return to your written piece. Did you use a reflective model to help structure your thoughts? Consider how use of a model could facilitate structured reflection of your own thoughts and how it could be used to explore practice with a student.

Portfolio development to demonstrate competence

Portfolio development has been a feature of some professions such as Arts and Architecture for a long time but became significant within the Health professions only in the early 1990s (Hull and Redfern, 1996; Pearce, 2003). This coincided with nursing education moving into higher education from an 'apprenticeship' style, 'training' type basis (Quinn and Hughes, 2007). Increasingly, the World Wide Web is influencing this area with e-portfolios and web logs (blogs) gaining popularity (Garrett and Jackson, 2006).

One principle associated with the use of portfolios stemmed from the fact that they provide the opportunity to demonstrate a more eclectic appreciation of the curriculum which not only focuses on skills development. To incorporate the broader, socio-economic, cultural and ethical dimensions of caring, portfolios offered the flexibility for individuals to be creative and selective in the evidence they supplied (Pearce, 2003).

The United Kingdom Central Council (UKCC, 1994 now NMC) also pronounced that all registered nurses should record their personal professional development by the maintenance of a portfolio. This was to demonstrate how they had updated their knowledge to remain eligible to seek re-registration on the professional register.

The Health Professions Council (HPC) endorses this view and has also incorporated portfolio development as a means of ensuring that their members continually update their knowledge and skills (HPC, 2006).

Portfolios have been adopted as a tool across professions to demonstrate personal growth and development. Various authors have noted that the act of developing the portfolio itself is an exercise that encourages skills of critical reflection and selection (Klenowski, 2002; Rae and Cook, 2000). When compiling them it is important to bear the audience in mind. There are different models that can provide a framework but again the fundamental consideration that drives the activity is who will read it and why are they looking at it? Types of evidence range from a simple collection of items to one that demonstrates progression to a high level of professional expertise, combined with a critical commentary on how that level of competence has been achieved. A portfolio may be viewed simply as a document containing details of what someone has achieved and can be assessed both formatively and summatively. However, this flat description does not encapsulate the living nature of a potentially very personal and exciting record of the experience and growth of a professional.

In a sense, a portfolio is never complete and it can be used to document lifelong learning which includes experiential learning from practice.

=============================== **ACTIVITY 6.4** ===============================

Consider your own portfolio. What sort of item does it contain? You may have had to adapt your portfolio for different situations, for example, academic courses where you have had to provide evidence of prior learning. Does your portfolio demonstrate your knowledge, skills and talent? What have you learned from portfolio development? Reflect on your experience of this and consider how your own knowledge could assist your student when developing their own portfolio.

Endacott *et al.* (2004) give a pragmatic description of different models that may be employed. These range from the basic idea of including a variety of evidence in a 'display case' format such as certificates, essays and so on that record education or training that the owner has undertaken. This is the simplest way of constructing the document and whilst it may identify good organisational skills and some creativity in design, it does not usually demonstrate intellectual or reasoning skills. They then suggest that the portfolio may be structured according to a specified format for a particular course or according to a pre-determined set of outcomes. This may contain documents such as reflective writing or witness statements that are linked and cross-referenced to the competencies.

However, the final model they suggest is that of a 'cake mix'. The analogy is useful as it relies on taking the evidence and then integrating it with the theory so that the narrative demonstrates the theory/practice link. This evidence can portray the individual's ability to manage more complex situations and maps the theory or research base that has guided their decision-making process. It captures the true essence of practice which is not always transparent to the observer and can contribute to the body of knowledge developed from experience.

When compiling a portfolio, it is crucial to be aware of the purpose of the exercise, as this will determine the management of it. Reflective accounts are an important part of a portfolio (Moon, 1999) and one way to review progress is revisit those written over a period of time to assess ones' development (McMullan *et al.* 2003). However, professionals do not always find reflective writing a valuable experience. Jasper (1999) explored nurses' perceptions on the value of written reflection; some found the process difficult and did not feel the need to write down their thoughts. Reflective pieces when used as part of a summative assessment may cause tension particularly for students who are caught between wanting to write about how they really feel and how they think they should feel to please their assessor. As Hargreaves (2004) states, students may be encouraged to suppress their thoughts and feelings in order to achieve a pass mark. Certainly self-disclosure can feel like a risky business although in a mutually trusting confidential relationship, it can be beneficial (Jack and Smith, 2007; Landeen *et al.* 1992).

The Practice Teacher has responsibility for providing placement experience for students to achieve the outcomes determined by the course curriculum. This can be difficult as the outcomes themselves may be non-specific and open to interpretation. Research undertaken by Scholes *et al.* (2004) indicated that practice assessors found the placement outcomes specified by the educational institution to be full of jargon and they stated that occasionally they lacked confidence in their understanding and interpretation of them. In fact, this was a distraction from the learning as the student and assessor were required to de-construct and then re-construct the outcomes around practice activities. The research also illuminated other concerns. Ultimately, the authors concluded that if portfolios are being used for assessment clear direction must be given as to the structure and content. The level of the learner should be borne in mind when the outcomes are written.

Portfolios are a common tool used for assessment whether formally towards a taught or work-based course, or more informally if preparing for an interview or documenting personal progress.

A good portfolio if demonstrating professional achievements must include robust links to theoretical reference points and provide examples of dynamic and proactive work. In order to demonstrate higher level cognitive skills an element of criticality should be included (Baume, 2003).

The navigation of this portfolio gives the reader an insight into the general organisational skills of the owner (Pearce, 2003). It can be frustrating if the reader cannot find evidence or if the evidence is poorly labelled or poorly explained. Therefore this chapter will conclude with some practical advice concerning how to compile a portfolio. When it is being presented in a particular forum then it may be necessary to edit it according to the context.

Remember that confidentiality must be maintained.

- The cover should be hardy, waterproof and personalised.

- A contents page and navigation tool at the front will enable the reader to find their way through the maze. This could also be cross-referenced to any specified outcomes.

- An index may also aid transparency.

- A rationale, explanation or information sheet could be placed at the beginning of the portfolio discussing the structure, content or any other relevant aspects of the development of the portfolio. This provides a context and will also focus the author's thoughts on why the portfolio is being created.

- A curriculum vitae

- A selection of appropriate evidence in the main body. Each piece of evidence should include a paragraph explaining the reason for its inclusion and be cross-referenced to any learning outcomes. It should also be accurately referenced.

Types of evidence

1. Evidence of attendance at study days: Certificates of attendance may be included in the portfolio but these alone are insufficient as evidence of learning. It is useful to write down and reflect on the learning gained and how this applies to practice. It is also useful to indicate areas for ongoing development.

2. Reflective accounts, significant events/critical incidents: Ghaye and Lillyman (2000) suggest an incident may range from an 'ordinary' experience to an incident that went well or was negative. However, despite the fact that the incident may appear trivial learning may still be achieved and that is what is important. A learning experience is a unique and personal event. Whist it can have significance for one individual it may not be of relevance to another, thus emphasising the personal nature of portfolios.

3. Continuous professional development materials and other interactive work-based articles/workbooks: These can be included within the portfolio to demonstrate specified learning on a particular subject. Many workbooks have 'time out' activities that can be used to evidence self-directed learning and development.

4. Formal assessment documents: These normally contain specified course outcomes which the learner has to meet to demonstrate practice competence. They follow a particular structure designed by the assessing institution. For example, key skills such as Information, Technology and Communication (ITC) skills can be mapped to the evidence compiled within the portfolio.

5. Learning contracts and action planning: These contracts form the foundation of portfolios developed for assessment purposes. They should clearly articulate the learning outcomes to be achieved and the action plan to accomplish this. They are a good source of evidence from which progression can be visibly observed.

Example of a learning contract based on communication skills

Learning outcome

At the conclusion of the placement, the student will be able to demonstrate interpersonal skills with patients/clients and their carers or significant others appropriate to their level of experience.

Action plan – using prompt questions to provide a focus

■ Where have I been?
Consider the prior learning and experience that the student brings with them. For example, the student may have prior experience as a waiter/ress dealing with difficult customers. This may mean that the student has some skills in managing confrontation. This could be a skill that is useful to transfer to the Health and Social Care setting. The Practice Teacher could discuss the student's previous experience with them and their perception of their learning needs.

■ Where am I going?
It is important that the student has a clear vision of what action is expected of them. It would not be natural for a student to manage a difficult therapeutic encounter without appropriate support and supervision in their first placement. The Practice Teacher is responsible for attending to the boundaries when facilitating the experience for the student.

■ How will I get there?
Think of the knowledge and skills that the student needs to develop and how this will be managed. It is vital to negotiate with the learner how this is to be achieved and assessed, ensuring that they are not threatened by the perceived enormity of the task. For example, this process may commence with the student observing the Practice Teacher acting as a role model during an episode which could then provide a vehicle for reflection.

■ How will I know when I have arrived?
The student should be aware of how they will be assessed in this outcome. Regular feedback is a feature of this process and also good facilitation to enable the student to voice their fears and anxieties. As Hull and Redfern, 1996 suggest it is important to create an environment in which the student can speak freely about his/her thoughts and feelings. This correlates with the idea of the 'practicum' described by Shardlow and Doel (1996) which is the provision of a sheltered environment for the student to test their skills and receive feedback.

================================ **ACTIVITY 6.5** ================================

Throughout this book there are different examples of learning contracts. Look at them and critically analyse them. Which one appeals to you and why? In preparation for the student you could create a learning contract as an example. This could be based on 'orientation to the placement' as this is a fundamental process required for all students. This could then be linked to a learning resource such as an induction pack.

Conclusion

It is paramount that the organisation has mechanisms in place to support Practice Teachers in their role. Thompson (2006) recommends that investment in this area can ultimately pay huge dividends by encouraging staff to examine how they operate and whether they could work more efficiently. Likewise, one aspect of clinical governance within the NHS relates to the use of supervision, the introduction of a 'no blame culture' but learning from mistakes through a process of reflection (DoH, 1999). Essentially the Practice Teacher is not working in isolation from the organisation. They must consider how to balance

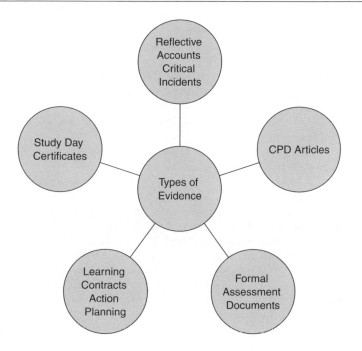

the priorities and pressures, ensuring that the student is not disadvantaged by extraneous issues.

Establishing the 'practicum' (Shardlow and Doel, 1996) in which the student can test their competence and skills in a protected environment will enable them to flourish in an atmosphere conducive to learning. Structured reflection is an inherent part of the process.

Reflective activity can establish whether the experiences that the student has encountered have aided their progression. How actively engaged the student has been and how their behaviour has changed can give a good indication of whether they have learned new knowledge and skills to build on the framework of their previous experience. The reflective process can provide a useful way of examining the student's progress. This chapter has provided a pragmatic view of how this may be achieved.

Resources

http://www.palgrave.com/skills4study/index.asp

This website offers a template with prompts that could be used to assist in writing a reflective diary.

http://www.businessballs.com/freepdfmaterials/reflective_diary_journal_templates.pdf

http://www.eportfolios.ac.uk/FDTL4/docs/fdtl4_docs/Cotterill_et_al_paper_for_eportfolios_2005.doc

References

Argyris, C. (1994) Good communication that blocks learning. *Harvard Business Review* July–August, 77–85.

Atkins, S. and Murphy, K. (1994) Reflective practice. *Nursing Standard* 8(39) 49–54.

Baume, D. (2003) *Supporting Portfolio Development.* York: Learning and Teaching Support Network.

Benner, P. (1984) *From Novice to Expert: Excellence and Power in Clinical Nursing Practice.* California: Addison–Wesley.

Benner P. and Tanner C. (1987) Clinical Judgement. How expert nurses use intuition. *American Journal of Nursing* 87(1), 23–31.

Boud, D., Keogh, R. and Walker, D. (1985) *Reflection: Turning Experience into Learning.* London: Kogan Page.

Boyd, E. and Fayles, A. (1983) Reflective learning: key to learning from experience. *Journal of Humanistic Psychology* 23(2) 99–117, cited in Powell J. (1989) The reflective practitioner in nursing. *Journal of Advanced Nursing* 14, 824–832.

Burnard, P. (2005) Reflections on reflection (Editorial). *Nurse Education Today* 25, 85–86.

Chimera, K. (2006) The use of reflective journals in the promotion of reflection and learning in post-registration nursing students. *Nurse Education Today* 27(3), 192–202.

Clegg, S., Tan, J. and Saedid, S. (2002) Reflecting or acting? Reflective practice and continuing professional development in higher education. *Reflective Practice* 2(1), 133–45.

Coutts-Jarman, J. (1993) Using reflection and experience in nurse education. *British Journal of Nursing* 2(1), 77–80.

Department of Health (1999) *Continuing Professional Development. Quality in the NHS.* London: HMSO.

Dewar, J. and Walker, E. (1999) Experiential learning: issues for supervision. *Journal of Advanced Nursing* 30(6), 1459–67.

Dewey, J. (1933) *How we think.* Boston: D. C. Heath cited in Coutts-Jarman, J. (1993) Using reflection and experience in nurse education. *British Journal of Nursing* 2(1), 77–80.

Doel, M. and Shardlow, S. (2005) *Modern Social Work Practice. Teaching and Learning in Practice Settings.* Aldershot: Ashgate.

Endacott, R., Gray, M., Jasper, M., McMullan, M., Miller, C., Scholes, J. and Webb, C. (2004) Using portfolios in the assessment of learning and competence; the impact of four models. *Nurse Education in Practice* 4, 250–7.

Faugier, J. (1994) The growth and support model. In Butterworth, T. and Faugier, J. (1994) *Clinical Supervision: A Position Paper.* Manchester: Manchester University.

Freshwater, D. and Stickley, T. (2004) The heart of the art: emotional intelligence in nurse education. *Nursing Inquiry* 11(2), 91–8.

Garrett, B. and Jackson, C. (2006) A mobile clinical e-portfolio for nursing and medical students, using wireless personal digital assistants (PDAs) *Nurse Education Today* 26(8), 647–54.

Ghaye, T. and Lillyman, S. (2000) *Reflection: Principles and Practice for Healthcare Professionals.* London: Quay Books.

Gibbs, G. (1988) *Learning by Doing: A Guide to Teaching and Learning Methods.* Oxford: Further Education Unit.

Haddock, J. (1997) Reflection in groups: contextual and theoretical considerations within nursing education and practice. *Nursing Education Today* 17, 381–5.

Hargreaves, J. (2004) So how do you feel about that? Assessing reflective practice. *Nurse Education Today* 24, 196–201.

Health Professions Council (2006) *Your Guide to our Standards for Continuing Professional Development.* London: HPC.

Heron, J. (1990) *Helping the Client: A Creative Practical Guide.* London: Sage.

Hull, C. and Redfern, L. (1996) *Profiles and Portfolios.* London: MacMillan.

Jack, K. and Smith, A. (2007) Promoting Self-awareness in nursing practice. *Nursing Standard* 21(32), 47–52.

Jarvis, P. (1992) Reflective practice and nursing. *Nurse Education Today* 12, 174–81.

Jasper, M. (1999) Nurses perceptions of the value of written reflection. *Nurse Education Today* 19, 452–63.

Jones, P.R. (1995) Hindsight bias in reflective practice; an empirical investigation. *Journal of Advanced Nursing* 21, 783–8.

Klenowski, V. (2002) *Developing Portfolios for Learning and Assessment. Processes and Principles.* London: Routledge Falmer.

Kolb, D. (1984) *Experiential Learning* London: Prentice Hall.

Landeen, J., Byrne, C. and Brown, B. (1992) Journal keeping as an educational strategy in teaching psychiatric nurses. *Journal of Advanced Nursing* 17, 347–55.

Mezirow, J. (1981) A critical theory of adult learning and education. *Adult Education* 32(1), 3–24.

Moon, J. (1999) *Reflection in Learning and Professional Development Theory and Practice.* London: Kogan Page.

McMullan, M., Endacott, R., Gray, M.A., Jasper, M., Miller, C.M.L., Scholes, J. and Webb, C. (2003) Portfolios and assessment of competence: a review of the literature. *Journal of Advanced Nursing* 41, 283–94.

Newell, R. (1992) Anxiety, accuracy and reflection: the limits of professional development. *Journal of Advanced Nursing* 17(11), 1326–33.

Nursing and Midwifery Council (2006) *Standards to Support Learning and Assessment in Practice: NMC Standards For Mentors, Practice Teachers and Teachers.* London: NMC.

Nursing and Midwifery Council (2008) *The Code: Standards of Conduct, Performance and Ethics for Nurses* London: NMC.

Paget, T. (2001) Reflective practice and clinical outcomes: practitioners' views on how reflective practice has influenced their clinical practice. *Journal of Clinical Nursing* 10, 204–14

Palmer, A., Burns, S. and Bulman, C. (1994) *Reflective Practice in Nursing: The Growth Of The Professional Practitioner.* London: Blackwell Science.

Pearce, R. (2003) *Profiles and Portfolios of Evidence,* Cheltenham: Nelson Thornes,

Quinn, F. and Hughes, S. (2007) *Principles and Practice of Nurse Education.* 5th edn. Cheltenham: Nelson Thornes.

Rae, K. and Cook, L. (2000) The portfolio experience: more than just a paper exercise. *Primary Health Care* 10 (7), 38–41.

Rolfe, G. (2001) Reflective practice: where now? *Nurse Education in Practice* 2, 21–9.

Shardlow, S. and Doel, M. (1996) *Practice Learning and Teaching.* Basingstoke: MacMillan Press.

Scholes, J., Webb, C., Endacott, R., Miller, C., Jasper, M. and McMullan, M. (2004) Making portfolios work in practice. *Journal of Advanced Nursing* 46 (6), 593–603.

Schon, D. (1983) *The Reflective Practitioner.* London: Temple Smith.

Schon, D.A. (1987) *Educating the Reflective Practitioner.* San Francisco: Jossey-Bass.

Smith, A. and Jack, K. (2005) Reflective practice: a meaningful task for students. *Nursing Standard* 19 (26), 33–7.

Taylor, M. (1987) Self-directed learning: more than meets the observer's eye. In Boud, D. and Griffin, V. (eds), *Appreciating Adults Learning: from the Learners' Perspective.* London: Kogan Page.

Teekman, B. (2000) Exploring reflective thinking in nursing practice. *Journal of Advanced Nursing* 31, 1125–35.

Thompson, N. (2006) *Promoting Workplace Learning.* Bristol: BASW Policy Press.

Tripp, D. (1993) *Critical Incidents in Teaching: Developing Professional Judgement.* London: Routledge.

United Kingdom Central Council for Nurses, Midwives and Health Visitors (1994) *The Future of Professional Practice – the Council's Standards for Education and Practice Following Registration.* London: UKCC.

The Virtual Reality of Learning?
New Ways of Learning

Jo Skinner

CHAPTER OBJECTIVES

Aim

To explore the role of the Practice Teacher in embracing new ways of learning.

Learning outcomes

- Appraise learning and teaching methods and their suitability for particular students and contexts.
- Evaluate the Practice Teacher's role in selecting and using learning and teaching methods in different learning and practice contexts.
- Analyse the guiding principles for Practice Teachers and reflect on using selected learning and teaching methods.

The explosion of new technologies means that there has never been such a wide range of ways to learn. This is re-shaping not only access to information but also learning and teaching methods and thereby the roles of learners and teachers. E-learning and digital media appear to supplant the need for real-time teaching and traditional methods, being perceived as quicker, more cost-effective and efficient. At the same time, there is an increasing demand for practitioners who have high-order interpersonal skills and who are confident and competent in practice (Skills for Health, 2007).

The role of the teacher needs to be aligned to these new ways of learning. Indeed, teachers, wherever they are based or whatever methods they use, remain responsible for directing learning and determining progression towards professional competence. Approaches to learning and teaching, and the methods used to achieve competencies, will vary. Innovative ways of learning seem to offer greater benefits than traditional methods, particularly for learner independence and autonomy, which fits well in to a model of lifelong learning in professional practice.

Given such variety, how do teachers know they are selecting the best methods for the learning outcomes and competencies that must be achieved? This chapter seeks to address this question by examining the spectrum of methods available and how they may be used, especially in relation to practice. Some principles will be offered to guide Practice Teachers in selecting learning and teaching methods. There is a close relationship to the learning theories, reflective practice and assessment that are discussed in Chapters 5, 6, 7 and 8, respectively. Strengths and limitations will be outlined with some comparison to traditional approaches.

New learning methods and how may they be used

Learning and teaching method may be described as any tool that is used to enable learning. It is the means by which teachers may expose knowledge, skills and information as well as attitudes and context. In other words, each method is concerned with 'how' the message is conveyed and is carefully selected according to 'what' needs to be conveyed. There is an infinite variety

Table 7.1 Overview of learning and teaching methods

Traditional teaching methods *– mainly derived from real-time teaching in class or practice*	New methods of learning *– mainly web-based and derived from technological developments*
Reading, taking notes, questions and answers	Distance learning packs, E-books, Personal Digital Assistant (PDA)
Lectures, formal teaching	E-learning, Web-based lectures, M-learning
Group work, discussion, workshops	Bulletin boards, discussion groups (synchronous or asynchronous), digital media
Seminars	Video conferencing
PowerPoint presentations, overhead slides	Web pages, Portable Document Formats (PDFs)
Observation and rehearsal of practical skills in clinical settings or role play	Virtual reality environments, simulation exercises
Video	Interactive web-based materials
Reflective diary	Reflection
Case studies, action learning, problem and enquiry-based learning	Web-based gaming, action learning
Tutorials	E-mail tutorials
Reflective practice	Virtual reflective practice
Learning contract	

of methods – especially enhanced by new technologies – and they can be used purposefully and creatively to bring the 'what' and 'how' of learning together (Table 7.1).

What distinguishes an old method from a new one? At first glance it is broadly the use of current technologies that frees up the time and place of study. These seem to be more pragmatic solutions to a time- and cost-driven society and raise philosophical questions about the value placed on professional education.

On closer inspection there are many parallels between old and new methods and what is important is their fitness for purpose. For example, taking notes in lectures may be just as effective as downloading lecture notes from a virtual learning environment (VLE). The method is about what the student is supposed to gain from the learning, so different methods will suit different people and situations. However, methods must be integrated into the student's learning journey, starting with the individual's learning style (see Chapters 3 and 5). This requires forward planning and flexible thinking on behalf of teachers.

Methods themselves are neither good nor bad just more or less appropriate to the particular curriculum learning. Thus the teacher must be proactive in selecting methods as part of an overall learning plan – this may be a learning contract. While teachers may have their own tried and trusted methods, they need to be mindful that variety is also important in maintaining attention, anyone who has sat through serial presentations understands the term 'death by PowerPoint!' Using a range of methods enhances motivation and interest for students and teachers alike. Methods that engage the senses fully, for instance the use of colour, sound or animation, can impact on mood and contribute to making learning a more memorable and pleasurable experience. However avoidance of sensory overload is also important (Child, 2007) and the methods chosen must have a value beyond pure entertainment!

The acceptability of learning methods by students may be directly related to their individual learning styles or prior learning experiences, that is, preference for 'hands on' practical experience. Practice Teachers ignore this at their peril and it is easier to adapt methods in one-to-one teaching, compared with group teaching. Practice Teachers are uniquely placed to get to know their students' learning styles, observing them when learning from and in practice or applying theory to practice. Practice Teachers can adapt their methods to suit preferred learning styles, that is, concrete, abstract, reflective or divergent (Kolb, 1984).

ACTIVITY 7.1

In reading this chapter, you are using the most common learning and teaching method. Do you find this is an effective method for you? Is there any other method you would prefer? What would it look like? How does this reflect your own learning style?

Classifying learning and teaching methods

Given the variety and complexity of methods, it is not possible to cover all of them in depth here. It is essential to note that they relate to the learning theories. For ease of reference the methods will be grouped in three broad classifications according to their primary focus:

- Remote learning
- Real-time learning
- Blended learning

Table 7.2 Summary of strengths and limitations of new learning methods

Strengths	Limitations
Can be re-used	Need constant updating of materials and upgrades to hardware and software
May enhance motivation	One size fits all approach
Easier to control pace of learning	Rigid form of learning may be more difficult to adapt to individuals' learning styles
May use resources efficiently if designed for more than one subject area	May be problematic for some forms of learning disabilities, that is, dyslexia
Primary source of learning where student determines the time and place of learning	Design may take a long time piloting a year minimum
Reinforces existing learning	May be expensive to develop and maintain currency
Expands or deepens learning	Tracking students may be crude with insufficient data of students progress
Alternative learning experiences, for example, ill-health or lack of real-time experience available	Tracking cannot verify it is the students accessing the material
Tracking tools can be built into VLEs to monitor student usage	Technical problems and compatibility, internet speeds
Self-assessment or progression tools can be built in	Relies on some technical competence of student
Inter-professional learning – where practical difficulties are encountered may use online discussion	Less portable form access to power sources etc.
Builds student confidence	Potential health and safety risk – work station assessment
Develops technical skills	Costs of initial hardware, printing etc.
Student support available	Little opportunity for informal learning and attitudes may be difficult to gauge
Aligns more readily with assessments	
Addresses needs of students in remote and rural areas	
24-hour access to material	

There are overlaps between methods and all are useful for practice-based learning; their strengths and limitations are summarized in Table 7.2.

a) Remote learning

Remote learning covers a variety of methods and is characterised by students' ability to learn away from a traditional learning environment at a predetermined time. Learning occurs in a virtual space and time continuum and because 'Every student needs a place to learn ....' (Santy and Smith, 2007, p. 83). Clarke (2004) identifies place, time and pace as the distinguishing elements of e-learning but text-based distance and open learning programmes have used the same approach for 40 years – widening access to learning. New digital media technologies together with an expanded Internet have revolutionised the pace and scale of developments (see Table 7.3). However these approaches put more onus on the student to engage actively in learning. This action includes browsing, investigating, making choices and doing things (Leeder, 2005), like participating in synchronous online discussion groups. These forms may be perceived as more accessible and flexible but paradoxically easier and less rigorous, although Becker (2004) challenges this view.

Digital media

This is the generic term for all digital media applications (see Table 7.3). As they grow so does their acceptability as legitimate methods of learning, indeed they have been embraced relatively uncritically. This may be driven by some assumptions that they offer quicker and cheaper results, are preferable to real-time teaching and make good use of resources particularly staff time; however fuller evaluation is required.

E-learning

E-learning is described by Clark (2004, p. 22) as, '...a general term conveying many different learning approaches that have in common their use of information and communication technologies'. This includes different uses of digital media such as video clips used in a web-based VLE such as blackboard (Table 7.3) and increasingly extended through mobile learning or M-learning. But, Practice Teachers 'need to remain aware that e-learning is simply a tool and its effectiveness rests with the management abilities of both tutors and students' (Becker, 2004, p. 39).

Designing methods and content is key to ensuring that learning is not trivialised, for example, inappropriate use of Gaming. However, developing more sophisticated e-learning methods is expensive, time consuming and requires frequent maintenance which has led to major investment in the development of Reusable Learning Objects (RLOs) (Leeder, 2007). RLOs are interactive web-based resources founded on a single learning objective, for example, needle stick injuries. They are freely available to teachers, stored in repositories through creative common licenses, and will become increasingly invaluable to practice-based learning (Table 7.3) (Wharrad and Bath-Hextall, 2006).

Table 7.3 Examples of how some new learning methods can be used

Methods	Examples	Uses
General web-based learning		
■ Internet/world wide web	Internet service providers: Yahoo, BT Search Engines: Google, Internet explorer	View and download material on to own computer E-mail accounts Research any topic and access material available in a digital form but information is not vetted
■ Websites	http://www.dh.gov.uk http://www.npc.co.uk/index.htm http://www.npci.org.uk/ http://www.nes.scot.nhs.uk/prescribing/index.html http://www.flyingstart.scot.nhs.uk/	Specialist information presented in a number of web pages, managed by an individual or organisation, each site has a home page providing an overview
■ Telephony	Mobile phones: Calls and text messaging, PDPs, e.g. Blackberry	Messages delivered via group texts to re-enforce learning or group discussion: Games
Digital media formats		
■ Digital imagery	Digital cameras Webcams Music: iPods/MP3/Podcasts	Role play and feedback on skills e.g. IPL Video conferencing Downloaded music and images for storage and replay
■ Gaming	See Prescription Errors Challenge www.prescribing.info	Specialist interactive games that develop confidence, understanding and competence e.g. use feedback and scores
Tailored methods for particular subject areas and student groups		
■ Virtual learning environments	WebCT Blackboard WebLearn See www.blackboard.com	Internet access to a protected site where focussed learning takes place. Normally through a recognised education institution where teachers manage learning materials and communication systems.
■ Reusable learning objects	Centres of Excellence in Teaching and Learning (CETL) see www.rlo-cetl.ac.uk/rlos.htm see also Filter database www.filter.ac.uk/ HEAL repository www.healcentral.org/	Sophisticated interactive resources held in repositories; See CETL resource on Reflective Writing includes theory on reflective writing, a quiz on learning styles and video clips of students talking about their experiences of reflective writing Health Education Assets Library (HEAL)
■ Action learning sets	www.natpact.nhs.uk/cms/316.php	Problem solving based on real life situations via small interdisciplinary group meetings

b) Real-time Learning

Much of the critique of traditional methods is that they are teacher centred and may foster passive learning (Leeder, 2005) in controlling the what, how, when and where. Newer forms of teacher initiated real-time learning, include action learning, simulation, inter-professional learning and reflective practice. Real-time learning may have added value in fostering attitudes and identifying failing students quickly and may be more cost-effective. Practice-based learning with one-to-one supervision is highly prized by students, although problems can be insurmountable.

Action learning

Most new learning and teaching methods are supported by technology even if just e-mail, however one method that has gained ground in health and social care is Action Learning, particularly at more senior management levels (Castley and Steel, undated). This is something that Practice Teachers may consider establishing for senior practitioner programmes and even for their own development. Action

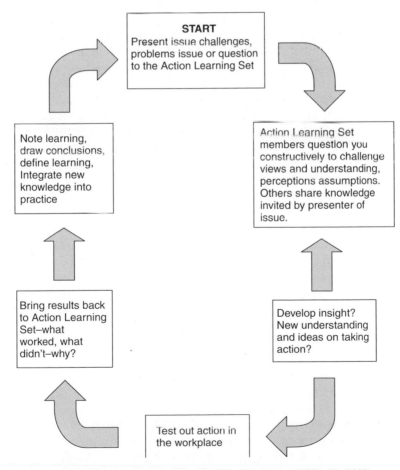

Figure 7.1 Action learning process adapted from NATPACT (2005)

learning involves small groups or sets (ALS) of participants meeting regularly to focus on individual or organisational issues to solve problems, develop learning and insight on the problem in order to effect change. Each ALS has a facilitator to enable staff to develop skills and work through group processes (see Figure 7.1).

Simulation

This method involves simulating real-life scenarios where students can develop and hone their skills using role play in a protected way. It is particularly useful for interpersonal skills fostering professional attitudes and inter-professional learning. The scenarios may be simple or elaborate, that is, from interviewing skills to a full-scale multi-disciplinary team meeting. This method suits most learning styles and can be useful for overcoming ethical concerns in practice. It can be used in assessment, such as Objective Structured Clinical Examinations (OSCEs), using actors. Simulation tends to be expensive and complex to set up, particularly if it is time sensitive.

Problem-based learning

This method is normally undertaken in small groups focussing on a real case or detailed scenario prepared in advance which provide problems which act as 'triggers' to stimulate learning. Students identify their own learning objectives and pursue the requisite knowledge and skills outside the group, returning with new knowledge having sought out the appropriate resources, including teachers (Price, 2003). The main purpose of this method is not merely solving the problem but facilitating richer learning and research skills as well as independence for individuals (Wood, 2003). Where there is a set curriculum, the objectives may well be pre-determined and has been used for many years in medical education. PBL works effectively for stable groups at the same stage in their programmes, with effective facilitation and where there is sufficient time and access to resources. It works best where the scenarios are sufficiently developed, relevant to immediate practice and are at the right level. Poor group working or weak independent learning skills will impact on the overall experience and outcomes. Practice Teachers can readily adopt this approach based on a case study of a patient or particular scenario providing guidance on discussion points through guided facilitation with clear objectives. PBL is particularly useful in building confidence in communication skills and team working in small groups. The Practice Teacher would need to judge carefully the stage the students were at as there may be uneven participation in the learning and assessing outcomes may be difficult.

Enquiry-based learning

Enquiry-based learning (EBL) is part of the family of student-centred approaches that includes action learning, PBL and individual projects. It is driven by students' motivation to learn, define and engage with problems in order to pursue solutions for themselves. It extends the ideas of PBL in that students generate their own questions, investigate and present solutions, leading to higher order thinking and the potential for originality through personal research (Kahn and O'Rourke, 2005). The teacher's role is key as a facilitator supplying triggers or scenarios, providing direction to resources and by developing students' ideas through supervision. Although this may traditionally be seen as a library based or independent research activity, it fits well with learning in and from practice. This is because not only does EBL relate closely to how adults learn and one-to-one teaching, but also because practice-based problems and enquiries tend to be complex and are naturally generated by the student. Students must also grapple with the practice solutions within an evidence based framework. Additionally EBL leads to deeper skills where students can tackle more complex issues, moving from novice to competence and onwards to proficiency and expertise. EBL also develops students' own leadership skills and may be particularly useful for postgraduate level programmes as it is intended to build on what students already know. However, this requires particular facilitation skills on the part of the PT and indeed restraint to prevent 'shutting down' lines of enquiry too early, providing 'unsound' solutions and further requires a level of confidence where new knowledge or evidence emerges that challenges the status quo.

Inter-professional learning

Inter-professional learning (IPL) has taken root as much as a philosophy of learning, influencing major curriculum re-design in health and social care, as a learning and teaching method. Evidence suggests that the earlier it is introduced into the curriculum the better the outcomes (Skinner and Pike, 1999). However, most IPL is classroom based, although the Common Learning in Practice (CLIP) model (Anthony, 2005) is a simple and opportunistic practice-based approach to IPL, allowing Practice Teachers to focus on common learning outcomes, joint learning experiences and mapping them into existing assessments.

Reflective practice

While reflective practice has been around for some time, it is being integrated into professional education to such an extent that 'being a reflective practitioner' is considered a norm by most professional bodies. The personal and experiential nature of practice-based learning lends itself well to reflective practice and acts '...as bridge between both mind and body and theory and practice...' (Salmon, 2006, p. 97). As reflection aids the development of critical faculties, from the Practice Teacher's perspective, it is both an important learning and teaching method and assessment method (Salmon, 2006). However, it also provides a challenge where a student's learning style is not reflective (reflection is discussed in greater depth in Chapter 6).

c) Blended learning

Blended learning denotes a mix of teaching modes: traditional classroom teaching, tutorials, online, electronic and practice-based learning. The 'blend' depends on what best fits the learning situation. New methods offer greater opportunities to stimulate, enhance and deepen learning by putting different approaches together, maximising student attainment. For instance, Clarke

(2004) asserts that the most successful online discussions are those that are initiated in real time. Blended learning is recommended for professional practice as it is unlikely that competence can be achieved using only one method or remote learning.

=================== ACTIVITY 7.2 ===================

Consider the following learning outcome and answer questions 1–3:

Learning outcome:

To assess a patient or client using an holistic assessment tool.

1. Select three learning and teaching methods you could use to achieve this outcome.
2. What are the limitations of each method?
3. How would you know you had selected the best method?

The Practice Teacher's role in relation to new methods

New methods challenge the assumptions of what learning is and what teaching is and also of each one's responsibility. Indeed, do we still need teachers or is it sufficient to have facilitated learning with a stronger role for teachers in assessing what has been learnt? Whilst accepting that adult learning and student autonomy are necessary, the Practice Teacher is responsible for setting the course of direction, clarifying what the final destination must be and defining staging points. In practical terms this means being familiar with the requirements of the programme and what is to be achieved in the time available and planning learning with students to achieve the outcomes. Practice Teachers will need to direct students to appropriate learning opportunities.

Learning contracts can be very helpful, and serve as a 'meta' learning and teaching method for the whole of practice-based learning, identifying not only what is to be learned by when, but also by what methods. Documenting learning plans, progress and achievements is an essential part of the role. The relationship between learning and teaching methods and assessment is important, so the Practice Teacher needs to align both to ensure students are adequately prepared. It is essential to have a strong communication strategy in place with students and the institutions.

For example, Table 7.4 shows a learning contract drawn up between the Practice Teacher and student, identifying the process for a student to become competent in undertaking a new assessment. The learning and teaching methods are ordered to allow, a logical progression of learning, a mix in self-directed, web-based learning, self and peer review, simulation and direct observation and supervision by the Practice Teacher and their relationship to the final assessment. This demonstrates a blended learning approach.

Table 7.4 Example of a learning contract

Learning outcome to be achieved	How learning outcome will be achieved	Assessment of competence	Progress review dates
Accurately assess a patient or client using an holistic assessment framework	• Fill out a blank assessment form based on data held in patient's or client's records		03.01.09
	• Download and read assessment tools and relevant protocols		10.01.09
	• Self-directed revision of interviewing technique using video		
	• Observe two new assessments with Practice Teacher		
	• Simulated new patient/client assessment with another student – peer review outcome		30.01.09 02.02.09
	• Undertake two supervised assessments		13.02.09
	• Complete one new assessment unsupervised		21.02.09
		Verified by client/ patient and PT observation of one new patient /client assessment by 06.03.09	

Professional values and curriculum issues

Practice Teachers will also need to balance professional requirements with those of the students. Programme approval and monitoring of the professional standards and competencies rests with statutory, regulatory and professional bodies. Practice Teachers need to ensure they are familiar with the standards as part of their overall accountability. Most professional bodies specify the role of practice and theory. Methods and assessments may be determined, for example, the balance of theory to practice and use of examinations; there will be flexibility for Practice Teachers to apply other methods to tackle the 'nitty gritty' of practice-based learning (Box 7.1). Professional values and standards can be very useful to explore the concepts of inter-professional learning and service user-centred care.

======== **ACTIVITY 7.3** ========

Reflection on values: How might a Practice Teacher help a student learn about the importance of involving service users in making decisions?

Supervision of practice is central to developing competencies but also for public protection as ethical standards of practice are integral to professional codes of practice. Methods used provide an important mechanism for highlighting professional values and standards of behaviour and practice. In particular, in practice-based learning, staff including Practice Teachers are powerful role models.

Box 7.1   Example showing how learning and teaching methods may be used to develop core values

A core value may be that service users ought to be central to decision-making. Methods that may convey this,

- Service users teach students in class
- Simulation or role play of service users making decisions
- Demonstration and observation of service users making decisions in practice
- Video of service users discussing merits of their involvement in decision-making followed by a guided discussion

Equity

Diversity and equity will also need to be considered (Forman *et al.* 2002), in practice this may be more difficult as the availability of practice experiences is unpredictable. Nonetheless, it can be planned for to ensure that there is equitable access to learning opportunities, for example, use of RLOs.

Students with disabilities require reasonable adjustments to be made so that students are not disadvantaged, in compliance with the Special Educational Needs and Disability Act (SENDA, 2001; DDA, 2005). The approved institutions have a primary responsibility here and will advise Practice Teachers. Students with statements identifying learning disabilities such as dyslexia, sensory or mobility problems require teachers to adapt existing learning and teaching methods and assessments. Typically, this means using different forms of the same methods, that is, adapting materials with different fonts, font size and colour; more time to read documents or complete tasks and physical adaptations to enhance access.

Guiding principles for Practice Teachers to select learning and teaching methods

Learning and teaching methods provide the opportunity to 'model' what we expect to see in students' outcomes. Therefore, the Practice Teacher's ability to select the most appropriate method is a critical part of planned learning to meet the learning outcomes and needs of the individual student as they relate to their preferred learning style and strengths.

Box 7.2 Principles for selecting a learning and teaching method

1. How does the method relate to the overall curriculum approach?
   e.g. A reflective approach may clash with one that requires precision, that is, numeracy.
2. Does the method allow the achievement of the learning outcome(s)?
   e.g. An interactive website may not match the practice learning skills to be mastered.
3. Does the method relate to required professional values or theoretical underpinnings?
   e.g. A student-centred approach is designed to mirror a client-centred approach.
4. Does the method fit the student's learning style or needs?
   e.g. A student who is a conceptual thinker may find an internet-based activity that must be followed in a set sequence restricting.
5. Is it clear how the method will help the student to learn?
   e.g. Selecting a new method may be counterproductive if it is more burdensome, that is, downloading large files rather than reading an article from a journal.
6. Is the learning method intended to foster active or passive learning?
   e.g. An interactive technology may not be pitched at the right level.
7. What other preparation or resources does this method need to be effective?
   e.g. All students have ready access to hardware/software and adequate time to complete tasks, supervision is available when necessary, SENDA compliant.
8. What other methods could be used to achieve the same result?
   e.g. The method is not the message – the ideas and skills need to be well managed through the method or else students may have to jump through many hoops to access them – such as precise direction to an active website or a focused discussion based on a real case study.
9. Why is this the best method?
   e.g. It supports efficient access to quality evidence or experiences available, up-to-date and relevant allowing competence to be developed and tested.
10. How will this method be evaluated?
    e.g. Identify in advance success criteria and a straightforward way of testing what works, that is, questions and answers, observation and evidence feedback is acted on.

Applying principles to practice

Box 7.2 shows a set of principles in the form of ten key questions that can be asked when selecting or evaluating learning and teaching methods, examples are given for each principle. Evaluation is central to the design of learning and teaching and there is evidence to suggest that it can be superficial and feedback is not acted upon (Adams and Skinner, 2001).

Implications of new learning methods for Practice Teachers

How knowledge is accessed, acquired and assimilated becomes blurred in the digital age with access to vast amounts of knowledge and information having been made open to the student. Discernment is required to select quality methods and web-based resources using the same skills needed for evidence-based practice (Upton, 1999), for example, how would a Practice Teacher use evidence from a Cochrane review compared with Wikepedia!

Tips for developing practice-based resources

- Set aside time to plan learning and own CPD
- Clarify programme level and student(s) skills and motivation
- Act on feedback from other students or staff
- Review access to equipment, IT support and upgrades
- Search for and appraise resources using evidence-based practice principles; exploit HE research e.g. Higher Education Academy
- Identify RLOs and websites that hold currency and relevance
- Request access to VLEs, resources used in class or web references
- Request and share resources with other Practice Teachers and HE colleagues
- Consider security, copyright and data protection and any license agreements
- Check when sites and resources were last updated
- Sustainability – don't assume online resources will exist for ever, save resources regularly
- Test resources first to determine areas of difficulty, allocating student time or if supplementary methods needed

================ **ACTIVITY 7.4** ================

Case study

You have a student with a known learning disability, dyslexia, who needs to develop his/her knowledge base of a common skill necessary for practice competence.

Work through the principles for selecting a learning and teaching method in Box 7.2 and consider:

1. What do you need to know about the curriculum the student is studying?
2. How will you plan their Learning Contract?
3. Which learning and teaching methods may be less suitable and why?
4. How might this impact on the final assessment?
5. How might you evaluate the success of your preferred method?

- Bookmark sources – request intranet space for PT
- Potential to establish own PT VLE for practice learning
- Devise methods of assessing effectiveness
- Evaluation strategy
- Review health and safety of learning environment ergonomics

Conclusion

This chapter explored the relative benefits of new methods of learning and place them in the context of educational theory and their application to professional practice and the role of the Practice Teacher. It is not a question of selecting to use old or new ways of learning but rather the one that best fits the learning situation and a blended learning approach is advocated as especially relevant for practice-based learning. The shift to self-directed and practice based-teaching continues and Practice Teachers need to be well prepared to use new ways of learning. The increasing emphasis on developing knowledge and skills to ensure competent practitioners who are fit for purpose is evident and this will include e-learning capabilities too.

Resources

Boud, D. and Feletti, G. (eds) (1997) The Challenge of Problem-based Learning, 2nd edn. London: Kogan Page.
Boyle, T. (1997) Design for Multimedia Learning. Hemel Hempstead: Prentice Hall.
Brookfield, S. (1998) Understanding and Facilitating Adult Learning. Milton Keynes: O.U.P.
Fry, H., Ketteridge, S. and Marshall, S. (eds) (1999) A Handbook for Teaching and Learning in Higher Education. London: Kogan Page.

References

Adams, N. and Skinner, J. (2001) *Evaluation: How to do it*. Primary Care Education Evaluation Project Funded by North London Education Consortium and Camden & Islington Health Authority.
Anthony, G. (2005) *Common Learning in Practice (CLIP) Inter-professional Placements Project Phase*. London: London Metropolitan University.
Becker, L. (2004) *How to Manage your Distance and Open Learning Course Palgrave Study Guides*. Basingstoke: Palgrave Macmillan.

Castley, A. and Steel, M. (Undated) Action Learning for Senior Managers: Addressing the Needs for Senior Management Development Using a Cross-institutional Initiative. [Online] *HESDA*, University of Sheffield. www.le.ac.uk/ua/sd/actionlearning/actionlearning.pdf (accessed 10 November 2007).

Child, D. (2007*) *Psychology and the Teacher,* 8th edn. New York: Continuum.

Clarke, A. (2004) *e-Learning Skills Palgrave Study Guides.* Basingstoke: Palgrave Macmillan.

Disability Discrimination Act. (2005) Disability Discrimination Act Factsheet: The Public Sector. [Online] http://www.dwp.gov.uk/aboutus/dda_factsheet2-public_bodies.pdf (accessed 3 January 2008).

Forman, D., Nyetanga, L. and Rich, T. (2002) E-learning and educational diversity. *Nurse Education Today* 22(1), 75–82.

Kahn, P. and O'Rourke, K. (2005) In Barret, T., Mac Labhrainn, I. and Fallon, H., Handbook of Enquiry and Problem Based Learning Galway: *CELT.* [Online] http://www.aishe.org/readings/2005-2/chapter1.pdf (accessed 3 January 2008).

Kolb, D. (1984) *Experiential Learning: Experience as a Source of Learning Development.* Englewood Cliffs, NJ: Prentice Hall.

Leeder, D. (2007) E-Learning Support for Interprofessional Education in Health & Social Care (ELSIE). *The Higher Education Academy Health Sciences and Practice Mini Projects* p.14.

Leeder, D. (2005) Re-usable Learning Objects in Practice Presentation to Universities' Collaboration in e-Learning at London Metropolitan University 22 March. [Online] http://www.londonmet.ac.uk/library/u23385_3.pdf (accessed 3 January 2008).

NATPACT (2005) [Online] http://www.natpact.nhs.uk/cms/316.php (3 January 2008).

Price, B. (2003) *Studying Nursing using Problem-based and Enquiry-based Learning.* London: Palgrave Macmillan.

Salmon, R. (2006) Assessing reflective learning: precepts, percepts and practice. *Investigations in University Teaching and Learning* 4 (01) Autumn, 97–104 Centre for Academic and Professional Development London Metropolitan University.

SENDA (2001) Special Educational Needs and Disability Act 2001 TSO. [Online] http://www.opsi.gov.uk/acts/acts2001/20010010.htm (accessed 3 January 2008).

Santy, J. and Smith, L. (2007) *Being an E-learner in Health and Social Care: A Student's Guide.* Oxon: Routledge.

Skills for Health Competences (2007) [Online] www.skillsforhealth.org.uk/page/competences (accessed 3 January 2008).

Skinner, J. and Pike, S. (1999) *Inter-professional Education and Working – A Scoping Study to Investigate the Development of An Inter-Professional Education Strategy in Primary Health Care* for the North London Education Consortium.

Upton, D. (1999) How can we achieve evidence-based practice if we have a theory–practice gap in nursing today? *Journal of Advanced Nursing* 29(3) 549–55.

Wharrad, H. and Bath-Hextall, F. (2006) Reusable Learning Objects in a Post-Resgistration Nurse Prescribing Courses (ROWEN). *The Higher Education Academy Health Sciences and Practice Mini Projects* p. 19. London: Health Sciences and Practice Subject Centre Health Academy Centre.

Wood, D.F. (2003) ABC of learning and teaching in medicine: problem based learning. *BMJ* 8 February, 326–30.

Principles of Assessment in Practice

Zoe Wilkes

CHAPTER OBJECTIVES

Aim

Critically explore the concepts and principles used in the process of assessing practice.

Learning outcomes

- Analyse the issues which affect the assessment of practice.
- Examine the role of the Practice Teacher in the assessment process.
- Propose strategies to strengthen objectivity in the assessment of practice.

Introduction

This chapter will examine the complex issues surrounding the outcome-based competency approach on the assessment of practice. Principles will be explored to determine how students' proficiency can be assessed at the point of registration, in order to ensure that as a qualified practical professional they will be able to apply evidence-based theory in a dynamic, clinical environment (HPC, 2004a, 2007a, 2007b; NMC, 2008). The concept of metacognition is introduced as an educational tool for Practice Teachers to use in developing and assessing transferable skills which practitioners can utilise in a variety of clinical settings to promote lawful, safe and effective future practice.

The purpose of assessment

The process of assessment is integral to teaching and learning and serves a variety of stakeholders (HPC, 2007a, 2007b; Manley and Garbett, 2000; UKCC, 1999). Assessment provides guidance and feedback for both the teacher and student and is generally described as a 'measure of achievement against a previously laid down standard' (Minton, 1997, p. 197). The Health Professions Council has a remit set by the Health Professions Order (2001, p. 4) to 'protect the public' by establishing 'standards of education, training conduct and performance for members of the relevant professions and to ensure maintenance of those standards'. Within programmes of nurse education, the professional regulating body, the Nursing and Midwifery Council fulfil this role to ensure that those applying to be placed on the professional register have achieved the required skills and knowledge to practice safely and effectively. The standards laid down by the Health Professions Council and Nursing and Midwifery Council provide a framework for learning outcomes which are used to measure achievement and establish proficiency at the point of registration.

The difficulties inherent in the assessment of practice apply to all practical professions and theorists can draw on the experiences of other disciplines (Ash and Phillips, 2000; Gonczi, 1994). Benner's (1984) work, frequently cited in nursing literature, applied the Dreyfus model (Dreyfus and Dreyfus, 1980) of skill acquisition to nurse education. Dreyfus and Dreyfus studied chess players and pilots and demonstrated that mastery of the skill led to a transition where smooth performance supported by analytical problem solving rendered the rules and formulae, learnt as a beginner, to the unconscious level. Furthermore, they observed that the performance of experts who were instructed to apply the basic rules deteriorated. Benners' (1984) continuum identified five stages of learning from novice to expert. She suggested that a competent practitioner can perform through the accomplishment of tasks to be competent in the role (third stage) but to become proficient and expert (fourth and fifth stage) the nurse had to make a 'leap'. Benner (1984) was criticised for her lack of scientific rationale and empiricism and demands for tighter definitions of words such as 'leap' were made based on objective measurement rather than hunches (Cash, 1995; English, 1993). Benner's continuum however does distinguish between accruing basic skills and holistic performance and as a tool it can enable teachers and students to understand the developmental process.

ACTIVITY 8.1

Reflect upon your own experiences of being assessed in practice. How was this achieved? Did the processes adequately assess what you had learned? Were you encouraged to develop your knowledge and skills further? Consider how these experiences can be explored and used to develop your own skills as an assessor.

The outcome-based competency approach to education

The assessment of competence was previously associated with National Vocational Qualification programmes and referred to the achievement of tasks or 'doing'. Despite the practical nature of many professions it was argued that this approach to education was reductionalist and simply 'doing' was not good enough for professions who needed to develop critical analysis and lifelong learning skills in their students (Girot, 2000; Watkins, 2000).

Competence as a concept created confusion as it was poorly defined and considered to be bureaucratic (Cowan *et al.* 2005; Girot, 2000; Watson *et al.* 2002); however the Peach Report, Fitness for Practice (UKCC, 1999), a comprehensive review of pre-qualifying nurse education, called for an outcome-based competency approach to nursing curricula. The report recognised the demands made on nurses to balance 'scientific rational and technical ability' within a holistic approach and suggested recommendations which identified the need to integrate practice and theory more closely. It argued that learning in the workplace was as valuable as academic learning and called for nurse educationalist and service providers to develop comprehensive definitions of competency and learning outcomes which facilitated learning and broadened the student's experience. This report was supported by the policy document 'Making a Difference' (DOH, 1999) and programmes of education were equally divided between a higher education institution (theory) and a clinical setting (practice placement).

The need to develop higher level competencies beyond basic skill acquisition was also being addressed by other practical professions (Ash and Phillips, 2000; Gonczi, 1994). A detailed exploration of competency by Manley and Garbett (2000) acknowledged the work of McClelland (1973) as the founding father of the competency movement. McClelland wanted to demonstrate that examination results were not the only form of assessment that could predict job performance or success as this method of assessment was biased against women and some ethnic groups. McClelland's research targeted practice-based disciplines and was able to link competency to effective performance not simply the acquisition of skills. Competency was associated with higher level skills in that if an individual could act 'intelligently and wisely' in different situations, it could be determined that they would do well in similar situations in the future. By returning to the source material Manley and Garbett (2000) have produced a grounded account of the competency-based approach to the assessment of practice which addresses the holistic aspects of the assessment of practice and provides a comprehensive summary.

> Competence is viewed as a person's ability to perform and their competencies as their total capability – what they can do, not necessarily what they do. Such competencies differentiate superior performance from average or poor performance by focusing on the person who does the job well – the characteristics and qualities that enable the person to do a superior job – rather than focusing on the job itself'. (Manley and Garbett, 2000, p. 349)

The literature distinguishes between competence and competency and suggests that the former refers to the individuals' ability to perform tasks whereas the latter (competency) focuses on the individual's performance which ensures the quality of patent care outcomes (Chapman, 1999; Manley and Garbett, 2000; McConnell, 2001; Woodruffe, 1993). This definition is further refined to competence as action and capability, competency as performance, person-orientated characteristics and qualities which referred to the behaviour of an individual underpinning their performance of the job (McMullen *et al.* 2003; Mustard, 2002). Capability therefore embraces competence but also identifies an individual's ability to apply cognitive and psychomotor skills to adapt to unfamiliar situations and environments while developing own performance and new knowledge (Fraser and Greenhalgh, 2001; NHS Education for Scotland, 2007; Watson, 2006). Educationalists therefore are challenged once again to ensure that practitioners are not only competent but also capable.

═══════════════ **ACTIVITY 8.2** ═══════════════

Reflect on definitions for the following: competence, competent, capability, proficient. How do these concepts overlap and how are they different? As an assessor how do you ensure that the student is both competent and capable at the end of their programme of study?

The complexity of assessing students in practice

The ongoing discussion of definitions demonstrates the complexity of assessing practice particularly at the point of registration when achievement of tasks is not enough to demonstrate proficiency. Consider, for example, the procedure of giving an injection. This is a simple procedure, a basic skill which can be taught to anyone. A proposal could be put forward to teach a milkman to give subcutaneous injections so that he/she would be able to attend diabetic patients in the community on his/her daily milk round. Indeed, the milkman could develop a strong business case for the job as the two services could be performed at the same time reducing the need for 'expensive community nurses'. In considering such a scenario the quintessential difference between a milkman, who may be competent, and a qualified nurse, who has competency and capability, identifies the component parts of nursing to determine how they are drawn together to create a professional practitioner fit for practice with professional values which are standards for action (Jormsri *et al.* 2005). Measuring basic competence or skill is relatively straightforward in that the student can either perform the skill or they cannot. Problems arise however when we try to assess the component skills which develop throughout the programme to create capability and achieve proficiency.

Educators recognise the difficulties involved in making the assessment of practice reliable, valid and objective (Chambers, 1998; Dolan, 2003; Gonczi, 1994; Milligan, 1998; Turner *et al.* 2003). Validity is concerned with the suitability of the assessment for measuring the attainment of the identified learning outcomes and reliability relates to the extent to which the outcomes are consistent (Quinn and Hughes, 2007). Any standard form of measure has to be reliable and valid, indeed Watson *et al.* (2002) insist that the assessment of practice must be 'accurately measured' but this could reduce the assessment of practice to measuring tasks and basic knowledge which demonstrates competence but not competency or capability. The reliability and validity of the assessment process is consequently called into question at this point as no reliable tool has been identified to measure proficiency (Nicol *et al.* 1996; Watson *et al.* 2002) despite many attempts to produce one (Chambers, 1998; Meretoja *et al.* 2004). The assessment of an individual's capability or performance requires the assessor to make a professional judgement which raises concerns about objectivity and Hager and Gonczi (1994) therefore argue that the strength or usefulness of the tool depends upon the person using it.

Assessing practice objectively as a Practice Teacher is further complicated by the conflicting demands within the role. A mentor is often defined broadly in the literature as a 'knowledgeable friend' (Bennett, 2002) and the process can be an informal arrangement developing a 'naturally formed' relationship offering lifelong support while promoting personal and professional development (Rose *et al.* 2005). Within health care however the Practice Teacher is allocated, not chosen and has responsibility for the assessment of the students' practice (AODP, 2006; NMC, 2008). This could present a dilemma as there may be tension between multiple roles and accountability.

Orland-Barak's (2002) study identified 'three selves' the mentor as a person who was genuinely concerned for the student and wanted them to do well, the mentor as a professional who had responsibility to maintain standards set by the professional regulating body and the mentor as a teacher who must assess student learning and determine whether learning outcomes have been achieved. The study suggested that this led to the feeling of being a 'mutant', a phrase which offers an accurate description of the conflicting emotions felt by mentors and Practice Teachers as they recognise their accountability to their profession, employer and teaching role. Feelings and emotions cannot be detached from the assessment process but must be managed to ensure that judgement is not affected and the assessment process is objective.

The problem of objectivity is not restricted to the assessment of practice. Yorke *et al.* (2000) analysed the spread of marks from six universities and found that the highest marks were awarded for Mathematics and Computer Sciences with Fine Art getting the lowest. When tutors were questioned about their approach to marking some insisted that they could recognise 'a performance' as achieving a certain level (percentage band). Marking schemes were used but there was a distinction between science-based subjects which were precise and the others (humanities) which required the tutor to make a 'judgement'. It appears therefore that only the assessment of empirical evidence or numerical data can be truly reliable and subjectivity will always be present to some degree (Chambers, 1998; Chapman, 1999; Dolan, 2003; Fordham, 2005; Gonczi, 1994; Manly and Garbett, 2000).

Demonstrating reliability and validity enhances objectivity within the assessment process but the art of assessment should not be restricted to a basic task-orientated process which avoids 'professional judgement' (Foster and Hawkins,

2004; Hager and Gonczi, 1994). Professional judgement is an integral part of the assessment of a profession and to dismiss it as lacking in validity and reliability trivialises the complexity of the assessment of practice and fail to capture the holistic nature of practical professions.

============================ **ACTIVITY 8.3** ============================

Reflect on a recent assessment you have undertaken with a student in practice. What criteria did you use to measure the student's performance? How objective was the assessment? Did you use your professional judgement to underpin your decision-making? How did you explicate your decision-making process?

The theory practice link

Ideally, when planning a curricula, educators should first identify the standard to be attained, develop learning objectives and align teaching and assessment strategies in order to determine when a student has achieved the objectives to the required standard (Hager and Gonczi, 1994; HPC, 2004b; Quinn and Hughes, 2007). Constructive alignment ensures that curriculum design effectively supports and measures student performance (Biggs, 1996). Therefore, in order to assess the practical capability of the student at the point of registration it is important to clarify what it is we are looking for.

Practitioners in health care today must translate concepts into action, develop systematic problem-solving approaches and discuss their rationale for decisions made whilst utilising scientific rationale, technical competence and providing holistic care (Bartles, 2005; Chapman, 1999; DOH, 1999; Fordham, 2005; HPC, 2004b; Koh, 2002). In order to achieve this balance between practical, technical and emotional ability practitioners must be able to integrate theory and practice to a level which goes beyond merely linking performance with cognitive processes (Ash and Phillips, 2000; Bassett, 2001; Dalton, 2005; Milligan, 1998; Pender and De Looy, 2004). To assess these diverse skills, values and knowledge in different practice environments assessment strategies must encompass a variety of techniques which draw on the same principles but can be tailored to align learning outcomes with student-centred learning and the demands of profession-specific practice.

The three domains of learning psychomotor, cognitive and affective are essential to the principles of outcome-based assessment (Reece and Walker, 2007). The psychomotor domain relates to practical skills which can be effectively assessed by observation and demonstration. Equally, the cognitive domain addresses knowledge and comprehension for which there are a variety of assessment tools which demonstrate reliability and validity. The affective domain however is concerned with feelings, commitment and values and gains importance throughout programmes of study in that the student internalises the skills and knowledge accrued to display behaviour consistent with professional standards (see Chapter 5 for further examination of these domains). This creates challenges for the assessment process in that attitudes and emotions are more difficult to measure with efficiency and objectivity but such complex behaviours must be assessed in order to ensure that practitioners can make an effective contribution to the development of the profession (Kuiper and Persut, 2004; Redfern *et al.* 2002). The process of metacognition is something we often do naturally but recent studies have indicated that the concept offers a potential strategy to transfer knowledge and skills into the required professional behaviour.

Cognition manifests in critical thinking and advanced reflection which is the key to metacognition. These skills satisfy several stakeholders in that they are sought by the professional regulatory bodies as standards to be achieved (HPC, 2004b, 2007a, 2007b; NMC 2004). They are of use to educators in that learning outcomes can be set and evaluated and are essential criteria for programmes of education (Kuiper and Persut, 2004). They are also valued by service providers as they support higher level decision-making and judgement required in the clinical setting and equip practitioners for lifelong learning (Kuiper, 2002).

Metacognition is generally associated with John Flavell (1977) a developmental psychologist and is commonly referred to as 'thinking about thinking' (Livingstong, 1997). Fontenyn and Cahill (1998) cite Paul (1993, p. 91) who neatly describe it as 'thinking about thinking in order to make your thinking better' but the concept of metacognition is more complicated than that (Kuiper and Persut, 2004; Veenman *et al.* 2006).

In order to facilitate the development of metacognitive skills students are encouraged by the teacher to reflect on and evaluate their activities which draws on the work of Vygotsky and Piaget (Kuhn and Dean, 2004; Martinez, 2006). 'Modelling' or talking a problem through with the student is advocated as a way of enabling a student to internalise the cognitive process but it is the meta-level which determines whether the student will continue to exercise this skill once supervision has ceased (Kuhn and Dean, 2004). Therefore, when a teacher 'thinks aloud' particularly during a difficult situation this cognitive thought process can be internalised by students (Martinez, 2006). Furthermore, if students are frequently asked questions such as 'Is that appropriate?' or 'How do you know?' or 'Why do you say that? they are more likely to ask these questions of themselves and implement the process of self-regulation which is the pervading theme associated with metacognition (Veenman *et al.* 2006).

The ability to develop metacognitive skills and knowledge appear to provide the distinction between the beginner and a competent, self-regulating practitioner who can be trusted to behave 'intelligently and wisely' hence 'safely and effectively' (Manley and Garbett, 2000). In order to develop metacognitive skills students must have the opportunity to practice them and be placed in situations in which they can be facilitated. The practice placement encourages the transfer of metacognitive strategies across various situations and ensures that the student is able to apply critical thinking in diverse clinical areas (Kupier, 2002). This ensures that the practitioner can adjust to changes in the practice environment demonstrating the required flexibility and adaptability characteristic in health care. The Practice Teacher therefore plays an essential part in developing the metacognitive strategies which can equip students for future practice. This relates back to the discussion about competence and capability. The preferred outcome is that the student is able to not only perform the requisite tasks to manage the presenting problem but is able to distinguish the complexities of the context in which this problem occurs and to respond appropriately. In this way they are demonstrating that they can adopt a holistic perspective by engaging higher levels of cognition.

============================ **ACTIVITY 8.4** ============================

Reflect on your own practice. Do you draw on metacognitive skills? List phrases or questions that you as a Practice Teacher could use to promote metacognitive skills in a student, for example, 'Talk me through your decision'.

Conclusion

The assessment of theory and practice are closely integrated and of equal worth. Objectivity in the assessment process will only be improved by collaborative working between educators, Practice Teachers and service providers. The progression from student to practitioner is dependent upon the ability to integrate classroom theory and skills with the reality of practice and the key to progression from the novice to the expert continuum is 'excellent mentor support' (Field, 2004). The concept of metacognition is worthy of further research as it is key to defining the difference between an average and a capable practitioner.

Resources

Foley, G. (2004) *Dimensions of Adult Learning. Adult Education and Training in a Global Era.* Maidenhead: OUP McGraw-Hill Education.
Bray, L. and Nettleton, P. Assessor or mentor? Role confusion in professional education. *Nurse Education Today* 27(8) 848–55.

References

AODP (2006) *Qualifications Framework for Mentors Supporting Learners in Practice: Standards and Guidance for Mentors and Practice Placements in Support of Pre-registration Diploma of Higher Education in Operating Department Practice Provision.* Cheshire: The Association of Operating Department Practitioners.
Ash, S. and Phillips, S. (2000) What is dietetic competence? Competency standards, competence and competency explained. *Australian Journal of Nutrition and Dietetics* 57(3) 147–51.
Bartles, J.E. (2005) Educating nurses for the 21st century. *Nursing and Health Sciences* 7, 221.
Bassett, C. (2001) Educating for care: A review of the literature. *Nurse Education in Practice* 1, 64–72.
Bennett, C. (2002) Making the most of mentorship. *Nursing Standard* 17(3), 29.
Benner, P. (1984) *From Novice to Expert. Excellence and Power in Clinical Nursing Practice.* California: Addison-Wesley Publishing Co.

Biggs, J. (1996) Enhancing teaching through constructive alignment. *Higher Education* 32 (3), 347–64.

Cash, P. (1995) Benner and expertise in nursing: a critique. *International Journal of Nursing Studies* 32(6), 527–34.

Chambers, M.A. (1998) Some issues in the assessment of clinical practice: a review of the literature. *Journal of Clinical Nursing* 7, 201–08.

Chapman, H. (1999) Some important limitations of competency-based education with respect to nurse education: an Australian perspective. *Nurse Education Today* 19, 129–35.

Cowan, D.T., Norman, I. and Coopamah, P. (2005) Competence in nursing practice: a controversial concept – A focused review of literature. *Nurse Education Today* 25(5), 355–62.

Dalton, G. (2005) Use of clinical space as an indicator of student nurse's professional development and changing need for support. *Nurse Education Today* 25(2), 126–31.

DOH (1999) *Making a Difference Strengthening the Nursing, Midwifery and Health Visiting Contribution to Health and Healthcare.* London: Department of Health.

Dolan, G. (2003) Assessing student nurse clinical competency: will we ever get it right? *Journal of Clinical Nursing* 12(1), 132–41.

Dreyfus, H.L. and Dreyfus S.E. (1980) Holism and hermeneutics. *Review of Metaphysics* 34, 3–23.

English, I. (1993) Intuition as a function of the expert nurse: a critique of Benner's novice to expert model. *Journal of Advanced Nursing* 18, 387–93.

Field, D.E. (2004) Moving from novice to expert-the value of learning in clinical practice: a literature review. *Nurse Education Today* 24(7), 560–5.

Flavell, J.H. (1977) *Cognitive Development.* New Jersey: Prentice-Hall.

Fonteyn, M.E. and Cahill, M. (1998) The use of clinical logs to improve nursing students metacognition: a pilot study. *Journal of Advanced Nursing* 28(1), 149–54.

Foster, T. and Hawkins, J. (2004) Performance of understanding. *Nurse Education Today* 24(5), 333–6.

Fordham, A.J. (2005) Using a competency based approach in nurse education. *Nursing Standard* 19(31), 41–8.

Fraser, S.W. and Greenhalgh, T. (2001) Coping with complexity: educating for capability. *British Medical Journal* 323(7316), 799–803.

Girot, E.A. (2000) Assessment of graduates and diplomats in practice in the U.K. – are we measuring the same level of competence? *Journal of Clinical Nursing* 9, 330–7.

Gonczi, A. (1994) Competency based assessment in the professions in Australia. *Assessment in Education: Principles Policy & Practice* 1(1), 27–42.

Hager, P. and Gonczi, A. (1994) General issues about assessment of competence. *Assessment and the Evaluation in Higher Education* 19(1), 3–14.

Health Professions Council (2001) *Health Professionals Order.* London: Health Professions Council.

Health Professions Council (2004a) *Standards of Proficiency. Operating Department Practitioners.* London: Health Professions Council.

Health Professions Council (2004b) *Standards of Education and Training.* London: Health Professions Council.

Health Professions Council (2007a) *Standards of Proficiency. Dieticians.* London: Health Professions Council.

Health Professions Council (2007b) *Standards of Proficiency. Paramedics.* London: Health Professions Council.

Jormsri, P., Kunaviktikul, W., Ketefian, S. and Chaowalit, A. (2005) Moral competence in nursing practice. *Nursing Ethics* 12(6), 582–94.

Koh, L.C. (2002) Practice-based teaching and nurse education. *Nursing Standard* 16(19), 38–42.

Kuiper, R.A. (2002) Enhancing metacognition through the reflective use of self-regulated learning strategies. *The Journal of Continuing Education in Nursing* 33(2), 78–87.

Kuiper, R.A. and Pesut, D.J. (2004) Promoting cognitive and metacognitive reflective skills in nursing practice: self-regulated learning theory. *Journal of Advanced Nursing* 45(4), 381–91.

Kuhn, D.E. and Dean, D. (2004) Metacognition: a bridge between cognitive psychology and educational practice. *Theory into Practice* Autumn 43(4), 268–73.

Livingston, J.A. (1997) *Metacognition: An Overview.* [Online] www.gse.buffalo.edu/fas/shuell/cep564/Metacog.htm (accessed 25 January 2008).

Manley, K. and Garbett, R. (2000) Paying Peter and Paul: reconciling concepts of expertise with competency for a clinical career structure. *Journal of Clinical Nursing* 9, 347–59.

Martinez, M.E. (2006) What is metacognition? *Phi Delta Kappan* 87(9), 696–9.

McClelland, D. (1973) Testing for competence rather than intelligence. In Manley, K. and Garbett, R. (2000) Paying Peter and Paul: reconciling concepts of expertise with competency for a clinical career structure. *Journal of Clinical Nursing* 9, 347–59.

McConnell, E.A. (2001) Competence vs. competency. *Nursing Management* 32(5).

McMullen, M., Endacott,R., Gray, M., Jasper, M.L., Scholes, C.J. and Webb, C. (2003) Portfolios and assessment of competence: a review of the literature. *Journal of Advanced Nursing* 41(3), 283–94.

Meretoja, R., Isoaho, H. and Leino-Kilp, H. (2004) Nurse competency scale: development and psychometric testing. *Journal of Advanced Nursing* 47(2), 124–33.

Mustard, L.W. (2002) Caring and competency. *Healthcare Law and Ethics* 4(2), 36–43.

Milligan, F. (1998) Defining and assessing competence: the distraction of outcomes and the importance of educational process. *Nurse Education Today* 18, 273–80.

Minton, D. (1997) *Teaching Skills in Further & Adult Education,* 2nd edn. London: Thomson.

NHS Education for Scotland. (2007) *Visible, Accessible and Integrated Care. A Capability Framework for Community Health Nursing.* Edinburgh: NHS Education for Scotland.

Nursing and Midwifery Council. (2004) *Standards for Proficiency for Pre-registration Nurse Education.* London: NMC.

Nursing and Midwifery Council. (2008) *Standards to Support Learning and Assessment in Practice.* London: NMC.

Nicol, M.J., Fox-Hiley, A., Bavin, C.J. and Sheg, R. (1996) Assessment of clinical and communication skills: operationalizing Benner's model. *Nurse Education Today* 16, 175–9.

Orland-Barak, L. (2002) What's in a case: what mentor's case reveal about the practice of mentoring. *Journal of Curriculum Studies* 34(4), 451–68.

Pender, F.T. and De Looy, A.E. (2004) Monitoring the development of clinical skills during training in the clinical placement. *Journal of Human Nutrition and Dietetics* 17, 25–54.

Quinn, F.M. and Hughes, S. (2007) *Principles and Practice of Nurse Education,* 5th edn. London: Nelson Thornes.

Redfern, S., Norman, I., Calman, L. Watson, R. and Murrells, T. (2002) Assessing competence to practice in nursing: a review of the literature. *Research Papers in Education* 17(1), 51–77.

Reece, I. and Walker, S. (2007) *Teaching, Training and Learning a Practical Guide,* 6th edn. Sunderland: Business Education Publishers.

Rose, G.L., Rukstalis, M.R. and Schuckit, M.A. (2005) Informal mentoring between faculty and medical students. *Journal of Medical Education,* 80(4), 344–8.

Turner, P. Doyle, C. and Hunt, L. A. (2003) Integrating practice into theory in the new nursing curriculum. *Nurse Education in Practice* 3(4), 228–35.

UKCC (1999) *Fitness for Practice. The UKCC Commission for Nursing and Midwifery Education.* London: United Kingdom Central Council.

UKCC (2001) *Fitness for Practice and Purpose. The Report of the UKCC's Post-Commission Development Group. Summary and Recommendations* London: United Kingdom Central Council.

Veenman, M.V.J., Van Hout-Wolters, B.H.A.M. and Afflerbach, P. (2006) Metacognition and learning: conceptual and methodological considerations *Metacognition and Learning* 1, 3–4.

Watkins, M.J. (2000) Competency for clinical practice. *Journal of Clinical Nursing* 9, 338–46.

Watson, R., Stimpson, A., Topping, A. and Porock, D. (2002) Clinical competence assessment in nursing: a systematic review of the literature. *Journal of Advanced Nursing* 39(5), 421–31.

Watson, R. (2006) Is there a role for higher education in preparing nurses? *Nurse Education Today,* 26(8), 622–6.

Woodruff, C. (1993) What is meant by competency? *Leadership and Organisational Development Journal* 14(1), 29–36.

Yorke, M., Bridges, P. and Woolfe, H. (2000) Mark distributions and marking in U.K. higher education. Some challenging issues. *Active Learning in Higher Education* 1(1), 7–27.

9

Methods of Assessment

Sally Hayes and Paul Mackreth

CHAPTER OBJECTIVES

Aim

To enable the Practice Teacher to undertake student assessment, ensuring that the student is assessed holistically utilising a variety of evidence-based assessment methods.

Learning outcomes

- Analyse and explain some of the key considerations when planning and taking part in student assessment.
- Produce and use an assessment method that is valid, reliable and feasible.
- Indicate transparent reasons for choosing a method of assessment.

Introduction

This chapter will build on the reader's knowledge of 'principles of assessment' to construct a working application of the methods of assessment in order to ensure fitness for practice in their students. This is not intended to be an exhaustive list of methods, nor seen as 'best practice' as every situation is different, but will aid the practitioner to develop a range of assessment tools.

Before examining the application of specific methods of assessment the purpose, complexity and challenge of ensuring that students are fit for practice both in today's health care setting and importantly for the future will be examined.

Assessment for learning

Several reasons to assess competence, including judging 'fitness to practice' are common to any learning situation: to direct and motivate learning; to ensure that correct standards are achieved before a student progresses to the next level; to provide feedback for students and also on the curriculum and method of delivery (Manogue *et al.* 2002). Careful planning and management is therefore required to ensure that the goal of 'professional status' can be achieved through assessment processes (Stuart, 2003).

The definition of assessment '... as a generic term for a set of processes that measures the outcomes of students' learning in terms of knowledge acquired, understanding developed, and skills gained' (Quality Assurance Agency for Higher Education, 2000) is arguably too simplistic as higher levels of learning concerns the process that the learner undertakes as well as the outcome of the learning.

Therefore assessment should not just be product focused in attaining a specific outcome, but also process-orientated in demonstrating the role of personal and professional growth (Price, 1994). This is key to the development of critical reflection – crucial to ensuring application of theory to practice (Moon, 2004) in a changing environment.

There is a plethora of academic writing on what needs to be considered and what follows is a distillation of this in order to give the reader an overview of what is important.

ACTIVITY 9.1

Before reading the following section of this chapter list out on a piece of paper at least five issues that you feel impact on the process of student assessment.

Subjectivity and objectivity

'There is enormous scope for subjectivity, especially when the competencies being assessed are relatively intangible ones to do with social and personal skills' McMullan *et al.* (2003, p. 287).

Assessment of clinical skills and performance relies heavily on observation, which by nature tends to be subjective and interpretations of performance may be inconsistent and unreliable (Stuart, 2003). The reliability of the assessment may be compromised by the differing standards of examiners, halo or millstone effects and racial or sex bias (Epstein and Hundert, 2002). As far as is possible therefore, subjectivity should be eliminated, and assessment carried out in ways where the grades or scores that students are awarded are independent of the assessor who happens to mark individual pieces of work. Students need to know what is expected of them; external examiners and moderators should be active contributors to assessment, rather than observers (Brown and Glasner, 1996) and where this is not possible the assessment criteria needs to be understandable, explicit and public.

Phillips *et al.* (1994) stated that there are two methods for looking at the issue of subjectivity of assessors' judgements regarding competence. The first is to make it as objective as possible, resulting in a long list of pre-specified skills to be ticked off to demonstrate that competence has been achieved. However, no assessment schedule can ever be assessor proof given the nature of interpretation. Alternatively, they advocate taking into account the subjectivity and also the assessor's perceptions and bias by making the assessment transparent to all involved in the process.

Other subjective issues that Hand (2006) describes may be physical or emotional factors affecting the students' performance – this may make them overtly nervous or clumsy during an assessment. This, he states, can be overcome through the use of a continuous assessment.

Hand (2006) further concludes that it is the very skill of the assessor to put this 'subjectivity' to one side through the development of self-awareness and honesty. If they cannot do this, then they need to consider their future role as an assessor. This issue is further explored in Chapter 3.

Validity and reliability

McMullan *et al.* (2003) highlight the importance of validity (that the assessment method measures what it is supposed to measure) and reliability (it measures this consistently). Despite this, in a study assessing practice of student nurse's (Calman *et al.* 2002), the students reported that tools gave far too little attention to psychomotor skill's leaving them with an anxiety about their ability to perform key skills. It was also noted that no institution had assessed the validity of competency assessment tools instead favouring student satisfaction evaluations.

Methods to overcome this could include using a set format of criteria for assessment. Such assessment instruments and processes need to be reliable and consistent (Brown and Glasner, 1996), but cannot be exact as assessors interpret things differently. Quality control must be used such as moderation by peers. In practice this could be achieved by the open discussion of ideas and concerns so that criteria and measurements can be changed and refined (Hand, 2006).

Torrance *et al.* (2005) however raise caution that the more transparent the method, criteria and usage of an assessment, then the more it can lead to 'instrumentalism', that is, the students succeed, but at what passing assessments? They state that learning should be a challenge and although students need coaching and an understanding of the assessment, it should still stretch their ability.

Learning styles

Assessment should be based on an understanding of how students learn and should play a positive role in the learning experiences of students (Brown and Glasner, 1996). One consideration here should therefore be learning styles.

A key study undertaken by the Learning and Skills Research Centre (Coffield *et al.* 2004) explored learning styles inventories and their pedagogical use. With over 71 models in use and background for commercial gain as well as theoretical and pedagogical activity they questioned their widespread use asking, 'if they are valid or reliable and what are the pedagogical implications'. The conclusions drawn are that assessors,

■ Need to be wary of some models in some situations.

■ Question the purpose of learning style models and match the correct model to the correct situation.

■ Ensure that they fully understand the background origin of the model.

They also found that the use of certain models could be expanded to assist teachers and teaching organisations to develop more student-centred and individualistic approaches to learning.

What are we measuring?

McMullan *et al.* (2003) explore issues of what is to be assessed and establish differences in the nature of competency. They conclude that it is the 'holistic' (i.e. knowledge, skills, values and attitudes) category of competence that best fits the world of a changing and dynamic practice arena. However, paradoxically it is this category of competence that is most difficult to assess. Therefore, they recommend that a breadth of assessment is required that utilises a multiple of differing assessment methods, that is, triangulation of the methods to gain a full picture; such as that which occurs during placement meetings between the Practice Teacher, lecturer and student (Mulholland *et al.* 2007).

Race (2005) argues that assessment tends to be governed by what is easy to assess and perhaps therefore not by what is important to measure. For example, how do you measure judgement, innovation and enterprise? However, in academic terms we must also ensure that the links between learning outcomes and assessment criteria are obvious to the students (Race, 2005). McMullan *et al.* (2003) discuss the impossibility of breaking down practice-based issues into criterion as it 'fragments' issues that then do not truly reflect practice and Gonczi *et al.* (1993 in Hand, 2006) reaffirms that competence involves more than performing a given task. Assessment is also about revealing the changes in cognitive, psychomotor and affective domain (Curzon, 1990). It is about ensuring that students have the correct knowledge, skills and attitude to practice and should not be done in isolation of practice, given that its aim is to assess just that. It is important, as theory and evidence should come from practice settings and therefore be about the 'real world'. This may only be achieved through continuous assessment methods (Hand, 2006).

In order to aid the Practice Teacher to 'pitch' the assessment to the correct level and expectation of a student, assistance can be gained from a variety of sources. One such source can be found from Covey (2004). His 'Maturity Continuum' can easily be adapted to student assessment.

Covey writes of developing self-awareness to aid the 'shift' of knowledge, skills and desire towards developing habitual character ethics of highly effective people. To do this he argues that a person must 'mature' through a continuum of dependence, independence to the final level of interdependence.

Likewise a student must be facilitated and assessed to develop knowledge skills and attitudes in a practice setting. Obviously, it would be unfair to assess a novice practitioner against criteria of interdependence. However, using the heading of interdependence, that is, a high level of maturity in a given area where the practitioner move from the 'I' of independence to the 'we' of interdependence (Covey, 2004), can also be a useful tool to allow practitioners to learn beyond their own level of competence.

Implications for practice

Assessment in itself should be a developmental activity, based on an understanding of how students learn and play a positive role in the learning experiences of students (Race, 2005).

Central to these concepts is the provision of feedback. Winning *et al.* (2006) noted that students reported a positive experience of assessment when the feedback they received was timely, constructive and detailed. They also appreciated feedback that gave strategies for improvement and encouraged them to further independent study. Students whose experience of assessment was negative commented on a lack of, or poor feedback. Feedback should therefore be timely, individual, empowering, encourage progress and be manageable for the teacher (Race, 2005).

Formative assessment – assessment which has a primary focus of feedback on achievement and does not count towards grades, is extremely useful to students in developing strategies to meet learning needs. It also offers rehearsal opportunities (Race, 2005). Even when summative forms (work that counts towards final grades) of assessment are employed, students should be provided with feedback on their performance, and information to help them identify where their strengths and weaknesses are.

Is it also very important to ask who assesses? Should it be self, service user, peer or team?

================= **ACTIVITY 9.2** =================

Think of at least one advantage and one disadvantage for the involvement of the following list of people in a student's assessment process.

- The student him/herself
- The service used
- The student's peers
- The wider clinical team

Self-assessment should be an ongoing process for students but formalising this in the use of student-developed learning contracts where the student is essentially setting his/her own development and assessment criteria is very useful. They can be used as an aid to critically reflective learning enabling students to deconstruct the learning outcomes of the course and examine how to further develop competencies (Moon, 2004).

In terms of service user assessment Wilkinson and Fontaine (2002) indicated how they were able to allow the patient rating of student competence which provided valuable information as to the 'whole' of the consultation and examination.

It is also important that there is diversity in the assessment process of a course to ensure that the same students are not repeatedly disadvantaged by the use of similar procedures (Race, 2005) and using a range of assessment techniques which promote motivation may also be helpful as student's levels of motivation and drivers are likely to change many times during a course (Iphofen, 1998).

It is therefore important that assessment is holistic and varied. Torrance *et al.* (2005) write of a 'smorgasbord' approach that is available for the assessor in a variety of different settings.

The remainder of this chapter will therefore be dedicated to exploring the 'smorgasbord' of possible assessment methods which can be applied in practice. It is not an exhaustive list but will consider the issues raised above.

ACTIVITY 9.3

On a separate piece of paper, write down as many different 'types' of assessment that you have been involved in. Consider these against the issues and implications discussed above. What (if any) changes could you make to your practice?

Assessment methods

Clinical competency profile

The 'Clinical Competency Profile' has become popular as a way of ensuring that practitioners have basic skill sets required to undertake a given role (DH, 1999). Competency, the ability of an individual (person orientated) and competence (job orientated) is what is required for a particular role or post (Manley and Garbett, 2000). The overall aim of assessment is the match of a practitioners 'competency' to a job role with required level of 'competence'. However, behind this lies complexity as literature abounds with the debate of what individual competency and role competence are (Hand, 2006).

Using the information detailed earlier in this chapter, the considerations for planners and assessors of clinical competency profile would be,

■ Does the competency profile accurately state what is required?

■ Does this clearly inform the student of the 'level' of performance?

■ Is the assessment of clinical competency about knowledge, skills, attitude or a combination of the three?

■ What number of individual competencies is reasonable to ensure validity but avoid over assessment?

If assessing areas of practice that are performed by 'expert' practitioners then the competency may involve the analysis of decision-making (Pratt *et al.* 2001). For example, exploring why an item was prescribed and what variables have been considered. However, if this is an assessment of a 'novice' such a Support Worker new to practice, then clearly higher levels of decision-making would be inappropriate. In its place would be the assessment of that which would ensure safety such as following a guideline, protocol or plan of care, that is, not attempting to make decisions in areas of uncertainty.

There are examples in areas of practice where clinical competency profiles have worked well (Myers, 2007). The accountability and responsibility of developing and delegating new skills for professionals and support workers requires a format that ensures that systems are in place to ensure due regard to these new roles. As Race (2005) contends, long lists can be counterproductive leading to a 'ticky boxy' approach (meaningless in the wider context of learning). Practice Teacher's will need to consider their approach to this method to ensure a positive learning environment.

Written assignment

A written assignment can be described as a traditional method of assessment and might not be expected to be seen in a chapter focusing on assessment in practice. However, Rolfe (1993) argues that there needs to be a clear and transparent link between practice and theoretical learning. This is important in preventing a theory–practice gap and ensures that learning is made real. Given this emphasis it is clear that Practice Teachers's should become involved in aspects of a student's written work, not as a marker but in ensuring the validity of the assignment task or aiding the moderation process.

The written assignment can also take a variety of forms to complement and augment learning in differing fields, for example, a time-constrained examination, dissertation, journal or a project/report. These tried and tested methods have clear advantages, not least that the student knows what to expect. Race (2005) adds that it

■ Allows for student individuality

■ Allows for demonstration of understanding of topic area

■ Assess writing style, a useful transferable skill

For the assessor, the written assignment is a manageable and feasible assessment format; however written assignments can be used with little consideration for the impact on learning in a field of practice. They can

■ Cause lack of equality as some students may never have been shown how to write essays well.

■ Be time consuming for staff to mark

■ Emphasise the 'halo effect'

■ Be time consuming for the student
(Adapted from Race, 2005)

It is therefore suggested that students are given assistance in essay writing by exhibiting examples of good and bad practice, that marking criteria are transparent, how the marks are allocated and word limits are clear if the question has several parts so students know what is expected of them. The latter promotes quality over quantity. Finally, relevant feedback should be offered and a statement of common mistakes used – this can minimise the time spent writing similar comments on different student essays.

Presentations

Visual and oral presentations may fit certain subject groups and situations and are useful as they have a rounded ability to assess both performance and content making the approach valid in today's contemporary health care setting (Brown and Pickford, 2006). In today's communication age students should be encouraged to use their own skills as an educator to develop competence in engaging learners.

Brown and Pickford (2006) highlight the ability to use presentations for learning:

■ Self-assessment

■ Audience assessment

■ Peer assessment

■ Team Presentations

The logistics of this form of assessment allow for almost instantaneous feedback which assists both students in developing learning strategies and the assessor as it is quick. However, the criteria for assessment needs careful planning, making much of the work for the assessor 'front loaded', in providing the student with clear outcomes to be met.

One example is poster presentation which utilise differing communication skills of students and demonstrate an important skill to aid employability, that is, meaningful learning with true vocational value. Summers (2005) experience of using this method to assess a cohort of School Nurses found many other positive attributes, including being positive in recognising student diversity. It allowed students who found the written word difficult, to express and truly reflect their ability to practice, for example, students with disabilities such as dyslexia. It also gave insight into values, experience of professional work and what is meaningful to students. She used the following criteria:

- Understanding of the audience
- Communication skills
- Evidenced-based practice
- Student development
- Analysis, synthesis and evaluation of knowledge

(Summers, 2005)

ACTIVITY 9.4

Reflect on what clinical competence could be assessed using a presentation. What are the strengths and weaknesses of this form of assessment?

Despite these positive attributes, her work highlights difficulties in summative assessment, such as feasibility with large student numbers and time for preparation, facilitation and presentation.

Objective Structured Clinical Examination

Objective Structured Clinical Examinations (OSCE) are described by Brown and Pickford (2006, p. 73) as, 'a series of stations where they [students] are asked to perform procedures. Assessment is via experts at each station'. The student's 'holistic' performance, can be assessed when undertaking the task including communication, interpersonal skills, problem solving and acting safely (Epstein and Hundert, 2002). This is achieved through a 'predetermined objective marking scheme' (Ward and Barratt, 2005).

Ward and Barratt (2005) further add that validity and reliability of the OSCE can be assured through careful planning, consultation, formative testing of the procedure to be assessed and the marking scheme. There is also an opportunity to gain patient feedback (Wilkinson and Fontaine, 2002) providing the opportunity to become 'patient' centred.

However, as with other assessments the temptation remains to break down the competency into smaller units, in the belief that mastery of individual components will indicate competency in the whole task. Performance descriptors specify functions and tasks, but not the knowledge, skills and attitudes underpinning them (Hager, 2004). The danger may be that students become competency driven, encouraged towards surface learning rather than a deeper, more holistic approach. It may be for this reason that the OSCE format has become adapted to Objective Structured Clinical Assessment (OSCA), which is a long-case scenario that follows a patient journey which can assess interaction and the level of professional ability in master's level thinking (Ward and Willis, 2006).

Resources are another key consideration (Alinier, 2003); they require the ability to work closely with a wide selection of experts and space for the stations and staff to manage the process. It is also the author's experience that the management of the planning and process is hugely complex. The OSCE has not yet reached its full potential however, over reliance on OSCE may limit our complete understanding of students' competence as it is difficult to reliably assess in the affective domain (Savage, 2006). As with all of the methods of assessment being discussed, it is important to use as part of portfolio of assessment.

Work-based study

A work-based study (WBS) is usually an extended study that examines the introduction of a new service or a review of an existing service, examining the underpinning theory and drivers and its application within the workplace. The focus is the development of practice within an organisational context (Flanagan *et al.* 2000). WBS should have definitive outcomes which can be evaluated relating to both service improvement and the competency of the individual practitioner leading these changes.

They are ideal assessment tools as the learning involved ie. learning by doing can be relevant to the students' work or future work experience. Learning contracts are negotiated with individual students as each project is different and allows students to demonstrate the integration of their learning in practice (Race, 2005).

They encourage the development of knowledge, critical understanding, practical and technical skills and professional attitudes and values through the negotiation required to achieve implementation and students gain skills in problem formulation, design and the generation and implementation of solutions (Flanagan *et al.* 2000).

The process can help demonstrate theory to practice, and policy to practice application, students learn time management and the employers (or future employers) can see the work-related competencies in addition to academic performance. It may also encourage employers to play an active part in student assessment (Race, 2005).

However as the project takes place in the workplace reliability is difficult and some students have better workplace opportunity to provide evidence of potential while others may be constrained into relatively routine work practices. They can also be time consuming for student and for supervisory and marking staff, and care must be taken to ensure that consistency of equity in practice is offered from each workplace or placement (Race, 2005).

Practice portfolio

A recurring theme of this chapter has been to ensure that a range of assessment methods are utilised to aid the holistic assessment. A portfolio is described as 'a purposeful collection of traditional and non-traditional work that represents a student's development and achievement over time' (Karlowisz, 2000). It can be suggested that this method of assessment is in itself holistic.

According to McMullan *et al.* (2003) the portfolio is popular as an assessment tool due to its congruence with Knowles (1990) assumptions of adult learners and Kolb's (1984) experiential learning cycle. They further indicate how professional groups see the portfolio as a method of integrating theory into practice, offering the opportunity to capture learning from experience, enabling an assessor to measure student outcomes. It also acts as a tool for reflective, analytical thinking and self-directed learning allowing the assessor to also assess the process of learning, (Scholes *et al.* 2004). This makes critical thinking and written reflections central to the development of portfolios (Moon, 2004)

The successful use of portfolios (Baume, 2001 in Scholes *et al.* 2004) however must be pitted against the insecurity that they can evoke in students who experience difficulties with the freedom of constructing an assessment with an un-prescribed structure. Measures should therefore be in place to prevent students' learning being distracted from their learning outcomes.

One measure is the construction of learning contracts within the development of the portfolio. This process enables the student to stop and consider (deconstruct) the learning outcomes of the course and construct aims and objectives which will address those learning outcomes. This is the point at which the theory–practice gap can be successfully bridged.

Portfolios give the student the opportunity to evidence their practice across a set time period. The process of self-assessment, key to portfolio development, is formative in addition to the portfolio being a summative tool. In this way portfolio development becomes a valuable learning experience.

Lecturers and Practice Teachers clearly need preparation to enable effective portfolio use by their students (Scholes *et al.* 2004). It is vital therefore that measures such as update days and regular meetings between students, course leaders and Practice Teacher's are maintained.

═══════════════════════ **ACTIVITY 9.5** ═══════════════════════

Think about the updates that you attend. Are you aware of the guidelines for assessment of students in practice? Who supports you in your role as a practice teacher?

At these meetings the authors find common areas for discussion, which are

- What is good evidence?

- The number of times pieces of evidence can be cross-referenced in order to keep the volume of the portfolio to a manageable size (Scholes *et al.* 2004).

- What is being assessed? The organisation of the evidence in the portfolio or confirmation that competence has been met.

- Should work be revised as the student progresses along the duration of the course?

- In enabling students to view their own progression by including in the portfolio early work, the overall final grade may be lower, or should progression be rewarded? That is, how far they have come (Scholes *et al.* 2004)?

■ Does it disengage students who struggle with writing reflective pieces?

It is important that all students being assessed by this means have clear and specific guidelines on how to construct their portfolio and have a shared understanding of the level expected of their work. It is good practice to show students relevant examples and suggest a proposed format, including suggesting a physical size. As portfolio building is usually time consuming, offer interim assessment opportunities so that students can receive advice on whether the evidence they are assembling is appropriate. An immediate source of knowledgeable support from the assessor should be available and the mentors/Practice Teachers need support (Scholes *et al.* 2004).

Conclusion

In conclusion, assessment should be viewed as a developmental activity based on an understanding of how students learn. It should be a positive learning experience for both student and assessor which encourage the exposure and examination of tacit knowledge through reflection promoting self-awareness and enabling practitioners (and assessors) to evaluate their practice (Jasper, 1999 in Scholes *et al.* 2004).

It must be acknowledged however that all forms of assessment have limitations, either for students or marking staff and care must be taken that it is appropriate to the desired outcomes for the individual student and the profession.

References

Alinier, G. (2003) Nursing students' and lecturers' perspectives of objective structured clinical examination incorporating simulation. Nurse Education Today 23, 419–26.

Brown, S. and Glasner, A. (eds), (1996) *500 Tips on Assessment*. London: Kogan Page.

Brown, S. and Pickford, R. (2006) *Assessing Skills and Practice*. London: Routledge.

Calman, L., Watson, R., Norman, I., Redfern, S. and Murrels, T. (2002) Assessing practice of student nurses. *Journal of Advanced nursing*, 38(5), 516–23.

Coffield, F., Moseley, D., Hall, E. and Ecclestone, K. (2004) *Should we be Using Learning Styles? What Research has to say to Practice*. London: Learning and Skills Research Centre.

Covey, S. (2004) *The Seven Habits of Highly Effective People*. London: Simon and Schuster.

Curzon, L. (1990) Teaching in Further Education. New York: Holt Rinehart and Winston.

Department of Health. (1999) *Making a Difference: Strengthening the Nursing, Midwifery and Health Visiting Contribution to Health and Healthcare*. London: The Stationary Office.

Epstein, R. and Hundert, E. (2002) Defining and assessing professional competence. *Journal of the American Medical Association* 287, 226–35.

Flanagan, J., Baldwin, S. and Clarke, D. (2000) Work-based learning as a means of developing and assessing nursing competence. *Journal of Clinical Nursing* 9(3), 360–8.

Hand, H. (2006) Assessment of learning in clinical practice. *Nursing Standard*, 21(4), 48–56.

Hager, P. (2004) The competence affair, or why vocational education and training urgently needs a new understanding of learning. *Journal of Vocational Education and Training* 56(3), 409–33.

Iphofen, R. (1998) Understanding motives in learning: mature students and learner responsibility. In Brown, S., Armstrong, S. and Thompson, G. (eds), *Motivating Students*. London: Kogan Page.

Karlowicz, K. (2000) The value of students portfolios to evaluate undergraduate nursing programmes. *Nurse Educator* 25, 82–7.

Knowles, M. (1990) *The Adult Learner: A Neglected Species*, 4th edn. Houston: Gulf Publishing.

Kolb, D.A. (1984) *Experiential Learning: Experience as the Source of Learning and Development*. London: Blackwell.

McMullan, M., Endacott, R., Gray, M., Jasper, M., Miller, C., Scholes, J. and Webb, C. (2003) Portfolios and assessment of competence: a review of the literature. *Journal of Advanced Nursing*, 41(3), 283–94.

Manley, K. and Garbett, B. (2000) Paying Peter and Paul: reconciling concepts of expertise with competency for clinical career structure. *Journal of Clinical Nursing*, 9, 347–59.

Manogue, M., Kelly, M., Bartakova Masaryk, S., Brown, G., Catalanotto, F., Choo-Soo, T., Delap, E., Godoroja, P., Morio, I., Rotgans, J. and Saag, M. (2002) Evolving methods of assessment. *European Journal of Dental Education*: 6(S3), 53–66.

Moon, J. (2004) *A Handbook of Reflective and Experiential Learning*. London: Routledge Falmer.

Mulholland, J., Mallik, M., Moran, P., Scammell, J. and Turnock, C. (2007) *Making Practice Based Learning Work: An Overview of the Nature of the Preparation of Practice Education in Five Health Care Disciplines*. [Online] http://www.health.heacademy.ac.uk/publications/occasionalpaper/occp6.pdf (accessed 18 December 2007).

Myers, D. (2007) Reviewing the support worker role in continence care. *Continence UK*, 1(1), 87–9.

Phillips, T., Bedford, H., Robinson, J. and Schostack, J. (1994), *Education, Dialogue and Assessment: Creating Partnership for Improving Practice*. London: English National Board for Nursing, Midwifery and Health Visiting.

Pratt, J.W., Raiffa, H. and Rchlaifer, R. (2001) *Introduction to Statistical Decision Theory*. London: MIT Press.

Price, A. (1994) Midwifery portfolios: making reflective records. *Modern Midwife*, 4, 35–8.

Quality Assurance Agency (2000) Code of Practice – Quality and Standards in HE [Online] *http://www.qaa.ac.uk/academicinfrastructure/codeOfPractice/fullintro.asp* (accessed 21 November 2001).

Race, P. (2005) *Making Learning Happen*. London: Sage.

Rolfe, G. (1993) Closing the theory–practice gap: a model of nursing praxis. *Journal of Clinical Nursing*, 2, 173–7.

Savage, J. (2006) In-training assessment (ITA): designing the whole to be more than the sum of the parts. *Medical Education:* 40, 13–16.

Scholes, J., Webb, C., Gray, M., Endacott, R., Miller, C., Jasper, M. and McMulan, M. (2004) Making portfolios work in practice. *Journal of Advanced nursing*, 46(6), 595–603.

Stuart, C. (2003) *Assessment, Supervision and Support in Clinical Practice*. Edinburgh: Churchill Livingstone.

Summers, K. (2005) Student assessment using poster presentations. Paediatric Nursing, 17(8), 24–6.

Torrance, H., Colley, H., Garratt, D., Jarvis, J., Piper, H., Ecclestone, K. and James, D. (2005) *The Impact of Different Modes of Assessment on Achievement and Progress in the Learning and Skills Sector*. London: Learning and Skills Research Centre.

Ward, H. and Barratt, J. (2005) Assessment of nurse practitioner advanced clinical practical skills: using the objective structured clinical examination (OSCE). *Primary Health Care* 15(10), 37–41.

Ward, H. and Willis, A. (2006) Assessing advanced clinical practical skills. *Primary Health Care,* 16(3), 22–4.

Wilkinson, T. and Fontaine, S. (2002) Patients' global ratings of student competence. Unreliable contamination or gold standard? *Medical Education,* 36, 1117–21.

Winning, T., Lim, E. and Townsend, G. (2006) Student Experiences of Assessment in Two Problem Based Dental Curricula: Adelaide and Dublin. Published for Australian Technology Network. [Online] http://0-journalsonline.tandf.co.uk.wam.leeds.ac (accessed 30 May 2007).

Managing Challenging Learning Situations

Sue Boran

CHAPTER OBJECTIVES

Aim

This chapter will explore the complex process involved in managing challenging situations in practice learning.

Learning outcomes

- Analyse the challenges adult learners face in higher education.
- Explore the complex relationship between student and Practice Teacher.
- Recognise students who are failing in practice.
- Appraise strategies and plans to address the issues.

The assessment of a student's practical ability in whatever setting has long been an integral part of any nurse or allied health professional's education programme leading to a recognised professional qualification. The importance of this is not only to ensure clinical competence but to guarantee patient and public safety, protection and confidence (Hand, 2003; Watson *et al.* 2002). The assessment of clinical practice has long been recognised as problematic (Watson *et al.* 2002) and the seminal research by Duffy (2003) on the subject of failing students has been useful in raising awareness of this complex subject.

Failing a student's clinical competency has been acknowledged as a very difficult thing to do and that it is inevitably influenced by personal, emotional as well as practical issues (Parker, 2003). Sharp's (2000) acknowledgment of the close one-to-one relationship between Practice Teacher and student in social work, reiterates that failing students can be a fraught, messy, emotional process that carries a threat of appeal and litigation.

Several authors allude to the fact that more students tend to fail the academic component than the practice part of their programme (Duffy, 2003; Scoles and Albarra, 2005) and that students are sometimes assessed as successful in practice when their performance is less than satisfactory, which is of great concern given the implications for both the profession and for client care and safety (Duffy, 2003). Some reasons have been put forward such as confusing assessment documentation, full of obscure, academic jargon (Duffy and Watson, 2001), insufficient time in placement to allow the student to develop competency (Watson and Harris, 1999), fragmented placement time which has not allowed continuity or that Practice Teachers have had insufficient time to work with students due to other pressing commitments on their roles in practice (Dolan, 2003).

It is also important to consider the student's perspective, particularly as throughout their education they are likely to come into contact with many professionals who influence the quality of their experience (Last and Fulbrook, 2003). Last and Fulbrook (2003) attempted to establish a consensus view of the reasons why student nurses leave their pre-registration education programme. With the exception of academic failure, there was no single contributing factor thought to make students leave, but issues such as communication and operational factors between the university and the clinical area, not feeling valued, unmet expectations and stress, were highlighted. The respondents in this study did agree that there was too much emphasis on the academic side of their education which resulted in a lack of confidence and influenced their level of knowledge of practical nursing skills. Students agreed that the high volume of academic work induces stress which inevitably impacts on their lives and inhibits their practical learning experience. This highlights the importance of communication between the educational establishment and the practice area to enhance understanding of the integration of theory and practice to ensure that most benefit is obtained for the student (DoH, 2000)

Challenges with learning

Gould *et al.* (2007), explored nurses experiences of continuing professional development, and found that the demands of undertaking study did encroach on life outside work, particularly home and domestic commitments and that these were perceived as barriers to achieving a desirable work-life balance. They identified factors such as time travelling to study events, arranging child care and accessing libraries and computing facilities outside working hours as important contributory factors as well as the amount of their own time that they were expected to contribute to their development. These are likely to be important considerations for part-time students particularly, as they balance work and study and potential financial deficits that studying may bring, especially as some students are expected to fund their own learning and use their own time to complete assignments. Norton *et al.* (1998) also commented on the variety of financial support mechanisms of mature students and Bryant (1995) found that a majority of mature students claim to encounter financial problems and that this has a negative effect on their studies. Cordell-Smith (2008) further supported this view.

For postgraduate students, the demands of studying at a more advanced level may be a challenge in itself, particularly if this is the first time that they are working at a level that demands wider reading and more in-depth critical analysis and synthesis of ideas.

Steele *et al.* (2005) also identified similar concerns from their work with mature students as well as relationship difficulties and the importance of coping mechanisms to overcome these problems such as support networks, prioritising and organising. Their work also highlighted the fact that mature students might have had very different experiences of education, which are dependent on gender, ethnicity, social class, marital status and the presence of school age children in the home. Seidler (cited in Steele *et al.* 2005) also found that men and women face different difficulties and situations in both educational experiences as well as their wider social situations.

Mature students have a number of roles and this can lead to conflict and tensions as they may need to renegotiate their gender-based roles as women are still seen as the natural carers of the home and children and have to manage the effect of course work on their domestic role (Steele *et al.* 2005). Anderson and Miezitis (1993) identified that female mature students used a range of coping mechanisms that include exercising, taking time out, coordinating schedules, changing one's thinking and communicating with family members, as well as utilising well-established coping strategies that they used prior to entering higher education. It is equally important for the student to negotiate with family members and friends the impact that their student role may have on their usual life.

When entering the learning environment many students might feel deskilled, or feel that they have been doing the job already and have the skills, knowledge and confidence to just 'get on with it'. Gould *et al.* (2007) agree that little has been written about the challenges faced by qualified nurses undertaking continuing professional development, despite the requirement to engage in lifelong learning and professional updating. This is where the Practice Teacher needs to be cautious. It is their role to act as a gatekeeper to the profession and to ensure that every student is competent to practice at this new level. It is often the case that practices have to be unlearned and relearned which can be a frustrating process for all concerned. It is the Practice Teacher's responsibility to protect the public and to ensure that the student operates effectively from a relevant evidence base. Practice Teachers in all health, allied health and social care professions have a critical role as gate-keepers for their professions. (Marsh *et al.* 2004). However, from a student perspective it can feel very frustrating when prior knowledge and experience is not acknowledged by the Practice Teacher. A study of post-registration nursing students showed that the change from qualified nurse to post-registration student can be unsettling both emotionally and through loss of status (Begley, 2006). The students became disillusioned when their prior qualifications and experience were not acknowledged. It is important to consider the academic and experiential journey taken by the student prior to arrival in the clinical setting. Practice Teachers can be challenged on aspects of practice about which they have little or no knowledge. It is useful to remember that students bring learning opportunities for the Practice Teacher and to use this to best advantage. Writing from a classroom perspective, Rogers (1996) describes the 'alternative expert' as a student who enjoys reminding the group that they have a lot of knowledge about a particular subject. In practice it is easy to understand why a student may want to demonstrate their ability by behaving in this way. In order to facilitate learning in practice, Practice Teachers need to be aware of their own limitations and understand how the student's strengths and background may contribute to the richness of the placement experience.

Cuthbertson *et al.* (2004) noted that there has been a policy-led drive to widen access to higher education and this has resulted in more mature students undertaking nurse education while Sparkes and Mason (2002), argue the need to widen access for mature students in physiotherapy. Mature students can bring with them valuable life skills and experiences which can help shape both their learning style and their ability to communicate with people. However, initiatives are not being adequately addressed and higher education institutes will have to develop much greater flexibility and innovative curricula to accommodate their needs.

ACTIVITY 10.1

Consider the particular influences on learning experienced by an adult learner.
How could you identify issues and support a learner who was experiencing particular challenges to productive learning?

Identifying unprofessional behaviour

Students are directed to their own unique code of conduct as well as other documents such as the Data Protection Act (1998), student disciplinary procedures, course handbooks and clinical and procedural policies that each health, allied health or social care agency provides in the placements. A student normally forms a contractual relationship with their higher education provider when they enrol (LSBU, 2007).

Unprofessional behaviour or professional unsuitability is demonstrated through any action or omission which could be judged to endanger public safety or bring the student, university or the profession into disrepute. Specific examples might include,

■ Failure to comply with their code of professional conduct.

■ Poor attendance and time keeping in the clinical or academic environment.

■ Consistent failure to communicate with the university or clinical placement which impacts on the associated clinical service delivery.

■ Failure to comply with professional guidelines and policies, such as dress code.

■ Failure to exercise due consideration for the safety and welfare of service users.

■ Failure to demonstrate consistent application to the development of professional skills (through appropriate interaction in the learning process).

■ Unacceptable behaviour in any environment.

■ Any action leading to a disciplinary procedure. (LSBU, 2005)

Many Practice Teachers will recognise areas for development in a student's performance, but that they do not constitute sufficient grounds for failure and many will only fail a student if 'unsafe' practice is demonstrated, such as inappropriate behaviour, cruelty, verbal and physical abuse and an abuse of the professional code of conduct. Other examples might include a lack of insight and knowledge of particular aspects of practice and yet students are still carrying out care, often to the detriment of the patient. Scanlon *et al.* (2001) have suggested that even though many examples of unsafe practice could be provided, the definition remains unclear and that few higher education institutions have clearly defined standards in relation to safe and unsafe clinical practice. Current assessment documents appear to have minimum standards; leaving it up to individuals to determine whether a student is actually unsafe (Duffy, 2003). It is essential to involve both the students' personal tutor and the educational institution if there is cause for concern.

It might also be useful for educational establishments to include learning outcomes with reference to professional behaviour and attitude within assessment documentation. This also encourages the debate around the perceived need for borderline status in clinical assessment (Duffy, 2003) a 'bottom line' in terms of level of competence (Skingley *et al.* 2007) and good enough practice to pass. However, the consequences of failing to fail have enormous implications and that the responsibility for this lies with Practice Teachers, managers and lecturers in a tripartite partnership approach.

Whether working in health, social care or in an allied health profession, the professional code is in place primarily to protect the public (GMC, 2006; HPC, 2004; NMC, 2008). A key component of this is acknowledging the limits of professional competence.

When addressing an issue with a learner in practice, a 'praise sandwich' approach can be useful. The Practice Teacher can begin by highlighting a positive aspect of the students' practice, then address the negative and finish with a positive (Hinchcliff, 1999). It can be useful to begin by asking the student how *they* feel the placement is progressing. Often the student will know that things aren't progressing smoothly and be glad to have the opportunity to raise the issue with the Practice Teacher. It is also very important to consider the timing of the discussions and the environment as it may not be a good idea to try and fit a meeting in at the end of a busy day, although the urgency of the situation may dictate this. Equally it would not be appropriate to have this sort of dialogue in a busy office where other members of staff can overhear.

Egan (1998) describes a three-stage model of helping which may be useful in this context:

- Explore the current situation with the learner. They need to understand what the issues are and they may be unaware that there is a problem. This is identification of the 'current scenario'.
- Identification of the preferred scenario. This will involve goal setting, to assist the learner to understand the 'preferred scenario'.
- This will involve an exploration of the ways in which the goals can be accomplished. This is the way that the learner can move from the 'current' to the 'preferred scenario'.

Conflict is a derivative of stress which is an indication that limits have been reached and are being felt. This is then expressed ideally in a conscious and respectful manner allowing the strengths and weaknesses to be discovered and understood. Discovery leads to creativity as new opportunities and changed dynamics become available and something new can occur or evolve because of this expanded understanding (Lebeck, 2003). Personality clashes may be blamed for work-based conflict although the issue may be a difference in learning style and a discussion of the difference in style could assist the situation (Cartney, 2004).

=============================== **ACTIVITY 10.2** ===============================

Reflect on a time when you had to give feedback to a student about an aspect of their work which needed developing. How and where did you do this? Think back to the event, were you aware of your body language, your tone of voice and what you said?

Mechanisms

It is good practice to identify formal progress points for assessment and ensure that these are understood by the student. Some of these may already be set by the higher education institute as formative and summative points on the students' programme. An initial meeting at the start of the placement could identify these points and should clearly document the methods and frequency of assessment and formulate an action plan. A mid-point assessment interview would also be useful in terms of documenting progress against programme outcomes, successes and areas for essential development before the end of the programme and a final interview would review the action plan and complete the assessment documentation. If meetings have been regular and recorded, this meeting should hold no surprises for the student. Long placements of perhaps a year would require more interim progress meetings for assessment (Marsh *et al.* 2004). It is crucial that students are given an opportunity to develop their practice following feedback from the Practice Teacher particularly if there are concerns (Parker, 2003). Failure of the placement should never be a complete shock to the student as assessment and feedback should have been ongoing. This approach is beneficial as it allows the student to consider their practice, discuss the constructive feedback presented by the Practice Teacher and to move on with a documented plan of action (Duffy, 2003). An action plan could identify short-term goals on areas that require development, with dates for review and how these might be achieved but also record what has been achieved towards the programme outcomes. Management of the situation may require support from others, for example, professional counselling or learning support if they are struggling with the academic demands of the programme.

Student learning can also be affected by other needs which the student does not have to declare. Provision of an environment in which the student feels safe and supported may encourage them to share any support needs they may have, for example, adapted equipment. If a student has developed a rapport with the Practice Teacher and the team and is happy to disclose their needs, then it is important to listen and discuss what would be beneficial to them, the team and client care (Stuart, 2007). Disclosure should be without fear of being discriminated against and in the United Kingdom, the Disability Discrimination Act (DDA, 1995) makes it an offence to discriminate against individuals for reason of their disability. In 2001, this act was further strengthened by the addition of the Special Educational Needs and Disability Act (SENDA, 2001). The Practice Teacher needs to be aware that students may have undiagnosed needs or even physical illness and sometime students struggle unknowingly for a long time before seeking support.

Sharp and Danbury (1999) emphasise the importance of collecting and documenting evidence when faced with a failing student as a clear, well-evidenced report will illustrate the decision-making process and will make it explicit where a student has failed to meet the competencies in practice. The Practice Teacher will need the support of their manager and should inform the educational establishment at the earliest opportunity if the student is requiring further support. Practice Teachers regard the support from lecturers as vital during difficult placements (Sharp and Danbury, 1999). All parties need to work together and respect decisions that are made.

Decisions made will inevitably be scrutinised by an examination board, which is why an accurate, clear and well-evidenced report is essential and support to write an appropriate report should be sought (Duffy, 2003). There is some evidence to suggest that lecturers and Practice Teachers should share the role of clinical assessor (Watson and Harris, 1999), or in the very least be present at any final meeting between Practice Teacher and student. This is by no means an established procedure and universities should have written protocols outlining the procedure to take in the event of a student who is failing in practice.

ACTIVITY 10.3

Consider your role as a Practice Teacher in terms of facilitating further support for students. Does your partner educational institution have a policy for supporting students? What systems are in place in your area to support Practice Teachers if they decide that the student has not met the outcomes in practice for a particular placement?

It should be recognised that providing intensive support is a time-consuming process and involves an increased workload for all concerned (Dolan, 2003; Phillips *et al.* 2000). For the lecturer this may necessitate extra placement visits within their current workload and for the Practice Teacher, additional time spent directly with the student in practice and regular, formal meetings to provide feedback for the student, will all place extra demands on time. However continuity of Practice Teacher is important so that they are able to provide an informed view of the issues. This fact is not necessarily recognised by immediate managers either in practice or in higher education (Duffy, 2003)

It is important to consider that failure of a practice placement may not always be a negative experience for a student. A student may be relieved that someone has made that decision for them, particularly if their chosen career pathway has not been what was expected or they are struggling and need to find a way out, yet they may not have had the courage to make that decision for themselves (Stuart, 2007). Indeed failure may prove to be a positive experience for some students who learn from the experience and go on to achieve success in another field.

Practice Teachers may be left with mixed emotions and dealing with the emotional aspects of a failing situation is not always something that they feel adequately prepared for. Many Practice Teacher educational preparation programmes will include sessions on managing challenging students, providing appropriate and timely feedback, dealing with emotional responses and record keeping (LSBU, 2005) and many higher education institutes also provide a series of support days for Practice Teachers who are assessing their students where this topic is often covered.

Practice Teachers need feedback on how they dealt with the situation and the final decision from the examination board, and it might be worth considering the need for a debriefing session between all concerned as a strategy following a failed clinical placement, in order to learn from the situation (Duffy, 2003)

Failure to fail is a common issue when faced with a weak student or leaving it too late in the placement before deciding to seek help (Duffy, 2003). The decision to fail is a big responsibility and could affect the student's career prospects in that they might be discontinued from their programme of study, which might be a reason for failing to fail. Other factors include consideration of the student's personal circumstances when considering the consequences of failing and as Scanlon (2001) recognises that failing could affect a student's financial situation, particularly for mature students, lone parents and those students who have caring responsibilities. This is very important, when considering the increasing numbers of non-traditional students entering higher education and the widening participation agenda. Watson (2006) defines widening participation as extending and enhancing access to higher education of people from under-represented backgrounds, groups and communities and positively enabling such people to participate and benefit from higher education. It is also concerned with diversity in terms of ethnicity, gender, disability and social background, including access across the age ranges.

Thompson (2003) reminds us that diversity is social variety across and within groups of people and is a positive attribute of the societies we live and work in. It should be seen as an asset to be affirmed and valued and not a problem to be solved. Equality of opportunity is based on a desire to achieve a fair starting point for people so that people are not disadvantaged in terms of access to employment, education and so on. A new approach that challenges this has come to be known as the diversity approach, which does not seek to replace equality as a focus of concern; rather that it has added another dimension to attempt to promote equality (Thompson, 2003). This new emphasis is on building positives in terms of valuing differences, not only in terms of gender and race or ethnicity, but also in relation to age and disability.

Conclusion

This chapter has explored the challenges faced by learners undertaking professional development and the complex relationship which exists between the learner and the Practice Teacher. It is important to recognise learners who need further support in order to be successful in their practical placement. Some learners will not meet the outcomes set and the Practice Teacher has a duty to make the decision to fail a learner. This can be a challenging time for the Practice Teacher and the need for robust record keeping and liaison with the higher education institute cannot be over emphasised.

References

Anderson, B.J. and Miezitis, S. (1993) Stress and life satisfaction in mature female graduate students. *Initiatives* 59 (1), 33–43.

Begley, T. (2006) Who am I now? The experience of being a post-registration children's student nurse in the first clinical placement. *Nurse Education Today* 27(5), 375–81.

Bryant, R. (1995) Why does being a mature student have to be so painful? *Adults Learning* 6(9), 270–1.

Cartney, P. (2004) How academic knowledge can support practice learning: a case study of learning styles. *Journal of Practice Teaching* 5(2), 51–72.

Cordell-Smith, R. (2008) Impact of debt on nursing students in higher education. *Nursing Standard* 22(19), 35–8.

Cuthbertson, P., Lauder, W., Steele, R., Cleary, S. and Bradshaw, J. (2004) A comparative study of the course-related family and financial problems of mature nursing students in Scotland and Australia. *Nurse Education Today* 24(5), 373–81.

Data Protection Act (1998). [Online] http://www.opsi.gov.uk/acts/acts1998/ukpga_19980029_en_1 (accessed 18 January 2008).

DDA (1995) *Disability Discrimination Act*. [Online] http://www.opsi.gov.uk/acts/acts1995/ukpga_19950050_en_1 (accessed 14 January 2008).

Department of Health (2000) *Placements in Focus*. London: English National Board, London.

Dolan, G. (2003) Assessing student nurse clinical competency: will we ever get it right? *Journal of Clinical Nursing* 12, 132–41.

Duffy, K. (2003) Failing Students: A Qualitative Study of the Factors That Influence the Decisions Regarding Assessment of a Students' Competence in Practice. Caledonian Nursing and Research Centre. (http://www.nmc-uk.org/aFrameDisplay.aspx?DocumentID=1330), accessed 4 June 2007.

Duffy, K., Watson, H.E. (2001) An interpretive study of the nurse teacher's role in practice placement areas. *Nurse Education Today* 21, 551–8.

Egan, G. (1998) *The Skilled Helper*, 6 edn. California Brooks Cole.

General Medical Council (2006) *Good Medical Practice*. London: GMC.

Gould, D., Drey, N. and Berridge, E.J. (2007) Nurses experience of continuing professional development. *Nurse Education Today* 27, 602–09.

Hand, H. (2003) The mentor's tale: a reflexive account of semi-structured interviews. *Nurse Researcher* 10(3), 15–27.

Health Professions Council (2004) *Standards of Conduct, Performance and Ethics*. London: HPC.

Hinchcliff, S. (1999) *The Practitioner as Teacher*, 2nd edn. Edinburgh: Bailliere Tindall.

Last, L. and Fulbrook, P. (2003) Why do student nurses leave? Suggestions from a Delphi study. *Nurse Education Today* 23(6), 449–58.

Lebeck, S. (2003). [Online] http://www.working-arts.com/stress-conflict-creativity_article.pdf (accessed 10 November 2007).

London South Bank University (2005) Directional Statement of Conduct Principles for Students of Nursing, Midwifery and Specialist Community Public Health Nursing (health visiting) at London: London South Bank University. LSBU.

London South Bank University (2007) Student Handbook. London: LSBU.

Marsh, S., Cooper, K., Jordan, G., Merrett, S., Scammell, J. and Clark, V. (2004) Assessment of Students in Health and Social Care: Managing Failing Students in Practice. Making Practice Based Learning Work. [Online] www.practicebasedlearning.org (accessed 4 June 2007).

Norton, L.S., Thomas, S., Morgan, K., Tilley, A. and Dickens, T.E. (1998) Full time studying and long term relationships: make or break for mature students. *British Journal of Guidance and Counselling* 26, 75–88.

Nursing and Midwifery Council (2008) *The Code: Standards of Conduct, Performance and Ethics For Nurses and Midwives*. London: NMC.

Parker, P. (2003) Assessment of Learning in Practice. In Glen, S. and Parker, P. (eds), *Supporting Learning in Nursing Practice; A Guide for Practitioners*. Basingstoke: Palgrave Macmillan.

Phillips, T., Schostak, J. and Tyler, J. (2000) *Practice and Assessment in Nursing and Midwifery: Doing it for Real*. London: English National Board for Nursing, Midwifery and Health Visiting.

Rogers, A. (1996) *Teaching Adults*. Buck: OUP.

Scanlon, J.M., Care, W.D. and Gessler, S. (2001) Dealing with the unsafe student in clinical practice. *Clinical Educator* 26(1), 23–7.

Scoles, J. and Albarra, J. (2005) Failure to fail: facing the consequences of inaction. *Nursing in Critical Care* 10(3), 113–15.

Seidler (1994) cited in Steele, R., Lauder, W., Caperchione, C. and Anastasi, J. (2005) An exploratory study of the concerns of mature access to nursing students and the coping strategies used to manage these adverse experiences. *Nurse Education Today* 25(7), 573–81.

SENDA (2001) Special Educational Needs and Disability Act. [Online] http://www.opsi.gov.uk/acts/acts2001/ukpga_20010010_en_1 (accessed 14 January 2008).

Sharp, M. (2000) The assessment of Incompetence: practice teachers' support needs when working with failing DipSW students. *Journal of Practice Teaching* 2(3), 5–18.

Sharp, M. and Danbury, H. (1999) *The Management of Failing DipSW Students*. Aldershot: Ashgate Publishing Limited.

Skingley, A., Arnott, J., Greaves, J. and Nabb, J. (2007) Supporting practice teachers to identify failing students. *British Journal of Community Nursing* 12(1), 28–32.

Sparkes, V.J. and Mason, C. (2002) Widening participation in physiotherapy education. Part 3: mature students in undergraduate education. *Physiotherapy* 88(5), 285–94.

Steele, R., Lauder, W., Caperchione, C. and Anastasi, J. (2005) An exploratory study of the concerns of mature access to nursing students and the coping strategies used to manage these adverse experiences. *Nurse Education Today* 25(7), 573–81.

Stuart, C. (2007) *Assessment, Supervision and Support in Clinical Practice: A Guide for Nurses, Midwives and Other Health Professionals.* 2nd edn. London: Churchill Livingstone.

Thompson, N. (2003) *Promoting Equality: Challenging Discrimination and Oppression,* 2nd edn. Basingstoke: Palgrave Macmillan.

Watson, D. (2006) *How to Think about Widening Participation in UK Higher Education.* A discussion paper for HEFCE. London: Institute of Education, University of London.

Watson, H.E. and Harris, B. (1999) *Supporting Students in Practice Placements in Scotland.* Glasgow: Glasgow Caledonian University: Department of Nursing and Community Health.

Watson, R., Stimpson, A., Topping, A. and Porock, D. (2002) Clinical competence assessment in nursing a systematic review of the literature. *Journal of Advanced Nursing* 39(5), 421–31.

11

Essentials of Evaluation

Pat Clarke and Heather McAskill

Evaluation has been described as the 'social science activity directed at collecting, analysing, interpreting and communicating information about the workings and effectiveness of social programs' (Rossi *et al.* 2004, p. 2). Alternatively, Jarvis and Gibson, 1997, p. 46) suggested it is an opportunity to examine the '... appropriateness of the aims, objectives and content and of the effectiveness and appropriateness of the methods employed'. It is also an opportunity for programme organisers to distinguish worthwhile methods of teaching/learning from those that are ineffective (Rossi *et al.* 2004). Therefore, evaluation can be regarded as a very complex and time-consuming process.

Evaluation has been recognised as an integral part of education effectiveness across the health and social care economies. Evaluation not only provides a tool for examining performance but also aids personal and professional development (Vuorinen *et al.* 2000). Furthermore, it can contribute towards the practice teachers' appraisal and identification of development needs (Neary, 2000; NMC, 2008).

It is important at this stage to differentiate between assessment and evaluation. There are numerous definitions of assessment as outlined in Chapters 8 and 9. Nicklin and Lankshear (2000) define assessment as a measurement that relates to the quantity and quality of learning and therefore is concerned with student progress and attainment. This is distinct from evaluation which is a systematic process of collecting, analysing, information about any aspect of educational programmes (Gopee, 2008; Mohanna *et al.* 2004).

Evaluation is a vital component of practice learning, providing an opportunity for Practice Teachers to identify whether the desired outcomes are being met, or identify if they are not. This has been reinforced within the new guidance for practice education published by the Nursing & Midwifery Council (NMC, 2008). Moreover, it is an integral part of practice education for allied health professions (Health Professions Council (HPC) 2007a). It is crucial to ensure that students' education is appropriate and relevant, ensuring that they are 'capable of safe and effective practice' (NMC, 2008, p. 13). It may also identify gaps in learning, enabling action plans to be put in place to address any issues raised, thereby providing a tool for ongoing improvement. The NMC requires systems to be in place for evaluating 'learning in practice and academic setting to ensure that the NMC standards of proficiency for registration ...' (2008, p. 54). This is similar to the requirements of the Health Professions Council.

Why evaluate?

There are numerous reasons for evaluation. For the financial year 2002/2003 the NHS spent £3 billion on education and training (Department of Health, 2002). Programme planners need to account how they spend tax payers' money, they must demonstrate public accountability, and evaluation can help to provide some of these answers.

The information generated from evaluation may provide some insight into the quality and effectiveness of practice learning and how the requirements of the NMC and HPC are being achieved (HPC, 2007a; NMC, 2008). Additionally, evaluation can provide evidence that the benchmark academic statements for health care subjects published by the Quality Assurance Agency (QAA) are being met. Outcomes from evaluation help to demonstrate accountability (Rossi *et al.* 2004). Indeed accountability and quality are inextricably linked. As health care educators we are accountable for the end product ensuring the student is 'fit for practice' and 'fit for purpose' (HPC, 2007b; NMC, 2008). Evaluation needs to be included in the validation documentation for any courses/programmes developed complying with both the requirements of the NMC and HPC (HPC, 2007a; NMC, 2008).

What do we need to evaluate?

There are many models and frameworks of evaluation that can contribute to a systematic approach (Gopee, 2008) and evaluators select models depending on the purpose of the evaluation. One of the most popular is Donabedian's (1988) model of quality assurance which focuses on the structure, process and outcome as components to evaluate learning. The evaluator may choose to evaluate only one component or use all three. Another approach used in education, particularly with the evaluation of programmes is the CIPP model which is an acronym for, context, input, process and product evaluation (Stufflebeam, 1971). Simplistically these four elements ask: What needs to be done? How should it be done? Is it being done? And did it succeed? Each of the four elements provided feedback on various components of a programme. These are often regarded as separate evaluations but like Donabedian they can be used as stages in a comprehensive evaluation.

However evaluation spans from a micro to macro level and Kirkpatrick's hierarchy four level model of evaluation illustrates this (Bates, 2004; Mohanna *et al.* 2004). Levels one, reaction and level two, learning, focuses on the individual, as opposed to level three and four, behaviour and result, which refer more to an organisational level and the impact on professional practice (Attree, 2006). The findings of an evaluation at a micro level can be used as evidence at each subsequent level finishing at the macro level. However, Kirkpatrick's four level pyramid model does not suggest that evaluation is a cyclical process.

Figure 11.1 outlines the phases of evaluation and that each stage can be interdependent on another or can be viewed in isolation. At a micro level it provides an opportunity to look at individual performance examining how students are facilitated and supported in the practice environment. Evaluation by self, student and peers are important elements of individual evaluation. On an advanced level evaluation can be undertaken relating to practice placements, requiring an increased level of organisation and co-ordination to complete (HPC, 2007a; NMC, 2008) and building upon the data collected at the individual levels of evaluation, that is, self, student and peer evaluation. Progression through the phases increases the complexity of evaluation. Moving onto a higher level might include programme and institutional evaluation. An example of this may be a university evaluating their programme of education. The final phase of this model could be seen as evaluation at a national level, such as that described using Ongoing Quality Monitor and Enhancement (OQME) (QAA, 2005).

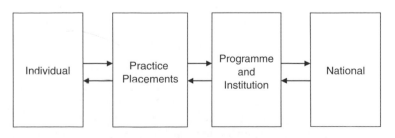

Figure 11.1 Phases of evaluation

Reflect on your current role as a Practice Teacher. What are the reasons for evaluation? Do you use any evaluation models to define the parameters of evaluation in your practice? Consider Figure 11.1 what is your role as Practice Teacher within each of the phases?

Individual

The micro level of evaluation focuses on the individual and is a measure of the quality of teaching. Performance indicators such as achievement by the learner of the learning outcomes can be considered as part of the evaluation process, however this assumes that quality teaching results in student learning and that poor quality teaching has a detrimental effect on student learning (Quinn and Hughes, 2007). The addition of other evaluation methods such as the use of self, peer or student assessment tools provides a more robust evaluation.

Self evaluation

It has been suggested that self evaluation is based on the Practice Teacher reflecting upon her practice and changing it accordingly (Gray, 2007). The NMC (2008, p. 20) suggested that the process of self evaluation can 'facilitate personal development, and contribute to the development of others'. It is acknowledged that the use of self evaluation to the exclusion of other sources of data may fail to provide a reliable comprehensive assessment of the Practice Teacher's development (Vuorinen *et al.* 2000). Setting standards too high can make self-assessment unrewarding. This could be due to the individual's own skills in self evaluation and ability to differentiate right from wrong answers (Dunning *et al.* 2003). In summary, there are some people who are unable to identify 'their own incompetence' (Dunning *et al.* 2003, p. 85) which may suggest that some of the data from self evaluation can be unreliable. Supporting the theory put forward by Dunning *et al.* (2003), Langendyk (2006) proposed the view that the over-rating of one's own ability can be the result of over confidence.

It can be challenging to establish a level of consistency in self evaluation because it is open to individual interpretation (Suls *et al.* 2002), and reliant on what the Practice Teacher wants to achieve from it. Stewart *et al.* (2000) put forward the view that self evaluation can be complicated and its outcomes can be affected by our own beliefs and norms. Self evaluation is also dependant on the practitioner's ability to reflect on her practice. Reflection will help the practitioner to develop an understanding of what is happening and consequently develop her practice, however there may be those who are challenged by this if they cannot decipher right from wrong (Dunning *et al.* 2003), finding it difficult to identify their own weaknesses as well as strengths. This may affect their whole understanding of the practice situation. As long as its limitations are acknowledged it may be able to form part of a wider evaluation but may provide inaccurate information if used in isolation. This is where the importance of self-awareness comes into effect as discussed in Chapter 3, and also

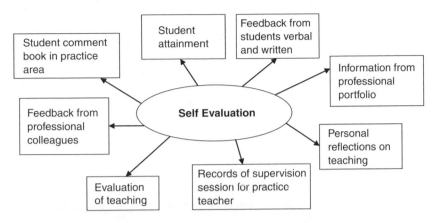

Figure 11.2 Types of information that may inform self evaluation

consideration of a variety of information to inform self evaluation as illustrated in Figure 11.2.

Alternatively peer evaluation provides the opportunity for Practice Teachers to collaborate and pool knowledge for reflection and discussion, enabling greater analysis of practice.

Peer evaluation

Peer evaluation has been described as '...a method by which the practitioner evaluates the work of a peer, according to set evaluation criteria' (Vuorinen *et al.* 2000, p. 273). Peer evaluation is integral to good practice and the evaluation process (Mohanna *et al.* 2004). According to Singh (2001) peer evaluation must be supported by an agreed framework such as guidelines and objectives. This formal approach would help organisations to adapt a consistent approach; however it may ignore individual needs Practice Teachers may wish to achieve through peer evaluation. A framework can provide quantifiable outcomes leaving it easier for organisations to justify investment in it. It is an important tool for Practice Teachers to use, to measure performance of their peers or be measured by their peers. Constructive feedback is a key element of peer evaluation (Vuorinen *et al.* 2000), without which no development can take place. Peer evaluation can provide a more in-depth measure of performance and it can build upon the outcomes of self evaluation. Moreover it helps the Practice Teacher to work collaboratively (Vuorinen *et al.* 2000).

One of the limitations of peer evaluation may be that the person undertaking the evaluation my feel uncomfortable being critical of a colleague, thus introducing bias into the process. The quality of peer evaluation may well depend on the insight of the Practice Teacher undertaking the peer evaluation into her own professional practice. Furthermore it can be time consuming in terms of the person undertaking the evaluation. On the other hand it may enhance her skills in self evaluation as well as assisting their own professional development. Like self evaluation, various types of information can contribute to peer evaluation (Figure 11.3).

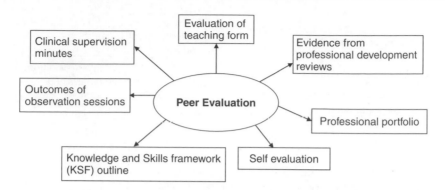

Figure 11.3   Types of Information that might inform peer evaluation

Student evaluation

One of the most important pieces of information used in evaluation is based on the outcomes of student ratings (Quinn and Hughes, 2007). Students can provide data at both an individual, placement and programme level. Like self and peer evaluation there are many methods to obtain information from students. Quantitative and qualitative information can be obtained through both verbal and written methods, the most common being a structured evaluation form. An example of an evaluation form that could be completed by a student, peer or oneself is illustrated in Table 11.1.

ACTIVITY 11.2

Reflect on evaluation forms you have previously used. Did the forms provide you with the required information? Can the same forms be used by students, peers and yourself to provide a depth of information? What variables do you need to consider when analysing the information? How do you know that you are evaluating your performance as a Practice Teacher? Did the information enable you to plan your development needs?

The Practice Teacher needs to be aware that responses from students may vary depending on the timing of the evaluation. The student may find it difficult to provide comments which could be deemed critical of the Practice Teacher. They may perceive this information as having an affect on their end of placement report. Furthermore, they may feel that negative feedback may have an impact on the student/Practice Teacher relationship. It must be recognised that some student feedback may be more reflective of their own difficulties within the placement than a realistic assessment of the learning experience (Phillips *et al.* 2000). Additionally, satisfaction with learning experiences can diminish overtime as students return to the workplace and find that the culture does not allow them implement their new knowledge from the course (Mohanna *et al.* 2004). Therefore, deciding on what to evaluate, using which indicator and when are integral to a reliable evaluation tool. The most comprehensive evaluation at an individual level would involve the

Table 11.1 Evaluation of teaching

Name:		Date:
Title of Session:		
Assessor:		

Structure	SCORE	
Poor introduction and no outline	1 2 3 4	Good introduction
Aims/outcomes not identified	1 2 3 4	Aims/outcomes clearly outlined
Inappropriate content	1 2 3 4	Content at appropriate level
Poor sequencing of material	1 2 3 4	Well linked, sequencing
Poor summary of session	1 2 3 4	Full conclusion outlined
Comments:		

Delivery

Appears poorly prepared	1 2 3 4	Well prepared
Monotonous and unclear voice	1 2 3 4	Varied speed and style of speech
Appears nervous	1 2 3 4	Confident and comfortable
Poor/inappropriate eye contact	1 2 3 4	Good/appropriate eye contact
Talked up/down to audience	1 2 3 4	Appropriate level of speech
Too long/short	1 2 3 4	Well timed
Poor student participation	1 2 3 4	Good student interaction
No check of learning	1 2 3 4	Evaluation of learning
Comments:		

Learning resources

Poor handling of relevant media	1 2 3 4	Effective use of relevant media
Poorly prepared/not legible	1 2 3 4	Well prepared and legible
Not suitable for subject matter	1 2 3 4	Suitable for subject matter
Inappropriate use of media	1 2 3 4	Media used to good effect
Comments:		

Question handling

Poor knowledge of subject	1 2 3 4	Good knowledge of subject
Poor questioning technique	1 2 3 4	Good questioning technique
Poor general impression	1 2 3 4	Excellent general impression
Comments:		
General comments:		
What were the strengths and weaknesses of the session?		
What are the recommendations for future development?		

Source: Adapted from Quinn and Hughes, 2007.

analysis of data from self, peer and student. This process mirrors the concept of 360 degree feedback.

360 degree feedback

The 360 degree feedback was originally developed for the business community as a staff development mechanism within the appraisal process, but more recently has been applied within educational and health care settings. The process has also been described as, multi-rater feedback, upward appraisal and multi-source evaluation. Although the names are different the concept is principally the same. Ward (1997, p. 4) defines 360 degree feedback as 'the systematic collection and feedback of performance data on an individual or group, derived from a number of the stakeholders in their performance'. Therefore, the key difference from traditional feedback is acknowledgement of the complexity of evaluation and that the use of multiple sources can help address some of the reliability factors.

Garbett *et al.* (2007) as part of an action research study to develop an accreditation process for clinical nursing expertise explored the use of a 360 degree feedback tool for peer review. The three recommendations from this study, to optimise the 360 degree process are useful to consider when evaluating practice teaching:

■ *Thorough preparation.* The purpose of the evaluation needs to be clear to all involved and the criteria for selecting individuals to participate needs to be evident.

■ *Suitability.* The approach to data collection needs to be appropriate. For example using a tool such as in Table 11.1 may be manageable but the detail of feedback may be less than using an interview.

■ *Anonymity.* Both open and anonymised approaches to collecting data are useful but need careful consideration, depending on the purpose of the evaluation. Open approaches can provide more constructive and detailed feedback for development.

While adopting the concept of 360 degree feedback in the evaluation process is considered as insightful in the development of the Practice Teacher, one must remember that it is only a component of the evaluation process. Inviting students and peers to provide feedback is not identical to a summative evaluation.

Placement evaluation

Placements are a crucial part of the overall learning experience (Cope *et al.* 2000) in health and social care as well as for allied health professionals and practice teaching is loosely linked to the quality of patient care (Gopee, 2008). In terms of nursing, practice comprises 50 per cent of the course (NMC, 2004) whereas social work diploma students require 130 days practice and 200 days practice for degree students (General Social Care Council (GSCC) 2006). The types of evidence that might be collected to complete an objective evaluation are illustrated as follows:

■ Outcomes of self evaluations

■ Outcomes of peer evaluations

■ Learning resources within the practice placement

- Evidence to support the quality of team working in the practice placement.

- Evidence of relationship between education provider and placement provider.

- Student module/placement evaluations

- Feedback from students

- Evidence of students achieving learning objectives for the placement

- Attendance of Practice Teachers at regular updates, and register of Practice Teachers

- Student reports

- Information from placement audits

- Reflective accounts

- Service user feedback

This provides a list of data which may be collected to support placement evaluation, however there may be other sources of documentation not mentioned above. The data derived from self, peer and student evaluation will provide crucial evidence for placement evaluation. Placement evaluation needs to incorporate information on placement arrangements and students' prior experience before the placement as this has been shown to have an impact on learning (Morris, 2007).

One of the key tools in evaluation is audit. The use of audit will help to provide information on the quality of education in practice learning environment (NMC, 2008) and '... determine, with others, audit criteria against which learning environments may be judged for their effectiveness in meeting NMC requirements' (NMC, 2008, p. 55). Auditing has been defined as '... a method of analysing what you do right, promoting what is done right and importantly, identifying what was wrong or what could be done better' (Cummins, 2006, p. 37). It will help to present a perspective on how practice relates to theory.

Information that is acquired through auditing can be used towards ongoing evaluation of practice learning, enabling practice to make ongoing improvements to the learning environment as referred to in Chapter 4. An example of audit might be examining whether the learning outcomes are being achieved within the placement. This type of data could contribute towards an evaluation of the learning environment. Furthermore, an audit of the supervision sessions between the student and Practice Teacher could also contribute to an evaluation of learning in practice. A further example of audit data that could be used as part of evaluation of practice learning could be record keeping audits. The audit would be able to measure if the Practice Teacher records were compliant with the NMC Record Keeping Guidelines (NMC, 2005) providing evidence of a direct link between theory and practice. It would also demonstrate how the Practice Teacher could be a role model for the student.

In addition, evidence collected to demonstrate compliance with Essence of Care Standards (Department of Health, 2001) could contribute to the evaluation of practice learning. 'Essence of Care benchmarking is a process of comparing, sharing and developing practice in order to achieve and sustain best practice' (Department of Health, 2003, p. 4). It is undertaken and owned by practitioners and it is their responsibility to develop practice using this framework. Where poor practice is identified the practitioners are required to put an action plan in place with deadlines to facilitate best practice to be achieved. Examples may include information about best practice achieved in relation to continence care, pressure ulcer care and nutrition. The aim of this is to ensure that wherever patients access the National Health Service they can be assured they will receive care that is considered 'best practice'. Consequently wherever students are training it was envisaged that their practical experience would also reflect 'best practice'. However because the interpretation of benchmarks was individual, information that may be used from this process to support evaluation of practice learning may lack validity.

It may be challenging and time consuming when trying to make sense of this amount of information, extracting only relevant data. Although where aims and objectives are outlined for the evaluation, data collected will be easier to analyse, because the collection of data will be more focussed. However the presence of aims and objectives may pose challenges in addressing unexpected issues that may arise in the data collected. The use of multiple sources of data can raise difficulties in reaching conclusions. An example of this might be that data from peer evaluation show the Practice Teacher as being effective in her role while the student evaluation of the module raises concerns about the placement and Practice Teacher; however it provides opportunities to identify problems and instigate actions plans to address problems identified.

ACTIVITY 11.3

Now consider what type of information you would collect to evaluate the effectiveness of your practice placement as a learning environment? Are there additional pieces of information that you feel would help to establish an objective evaluation?

Programme and institution evaluation

Programme evaluation helps to demonstrate the quality of a health and social care programme and needs to be separate from the evaluation of teaching as it includes characteristics such as organisation and resources. This process is now well established in higher education (Quinn and Hughes, 2007). Programme evaluation needs to examine the practical component as well as the academic component. This evaluation will build upon the outcomes of self, peer and placement evaluation. It will need to include information on stakeholders such as local employers. It has been acknowledged that education provision is more likely to be enhanced where there is visible external support (Swalfield and MacBeath, 2005). Indeed the Health Professions Council (2007a) suggested that it should include evidence from module evaluations, placement evaluation, programme committees and student liaison committees. This information will provide evidence to demonstrate that the programme is 'fit for purpose'. The evaluation needs to take account of support for students particularly those who are failing, in terms of how they are supported both in the academic component as well as practice. Additionally it should also include evidence on the effectiveness of assessments both practical and academic (NMC, 2008). The external examiner provides an objective perspective on this aspect of the programme, moderating student's work and ensuring that standards are comparable with other higher education institutions in the country.

=== **ACTIVITY 11.4** ===

Reflect on the programme that you support students on. Do you receive the outcomes of the evaluations? What processes are in place to allow you to contribute to the evaluation of the programme? How does the outcome of the programme evaluations enhance your role as a Practice Teacher?

Practice Teachers will probably not have much involvement with evaluation at an institutional level but should have an awareness of the salient issues of quality assurance at this level, such as programme monitoring and internal audits.

National level

Major Review and Ongoing Quality Monitoring and Enhancement (OQME) are examples of evaluation at a national level. These will be explored in more depth in Chapter 14.

The Practice Teacher can contribute valuable information to this evaluation. Examples include risk assessments which are required for students while on placement, outcomes of practice placement audits. In terms of monitoring visits organised by NMC, QAA and HPC the Practice Teacher can also provide 'rich' information about the quality of the relationship with the education provider, show the type of risk assessments completed in relation to students on practice placements. Moreover, she can provide evidence of the variety of learning resources available to the student. Indeed it could be said that the Practice Teacher is the key provider of information about the practice placement. The Practice Teacher may be asked for evidence to demonstrate how the organisation supports her with her ongoing development. Evidence to support this may include the policy on staff development. The Practice Teacher can also provide information regarding how issues are dealt with in the practice placement. The monitoring team can obtain information about how changes are made as a result of problems identified following placement audits.

Conclusion

Regular evaluation of practice teaching will help to ensure that the academic and practical components of the programme are 'Fit for Purpose' meeting the requirements of the changing health care setting (Rossi *et al.* 2004). Evaluation needs to contribute to improvement at an individual level as well as organisational level. Evaluation helps to move away from the 'change for change sake' culture to change based on evidence.

Clearly, evaluation is multi-faceted, so to analyse the effectiveness of practice learning, effective evaluation needs to incorporate not just one source of data but needs to take account of many sources to reach a balanced outcome.

As discussed in this chapter, evaluation can be a major exercise to ensure all aspects that could impact on practice learning are taken into account; hence it can be very costly in terms of time and resources. The depth and breadth of the evaluation may depend on individual organisation's priorities in relation to practice learning at that time. Dean (2000) put forward the view that the sustainability of the learning organisation may be dependant on the presence of evaluation to support and facilitate it to adjust to change.

Resources

CIPP Evaluation Model Checklist: http://www.wmich.edu/evalctr/checklists/cippchecklist.htm

Making Practice Based Learning Work: http://www.practicebasedlearning.org/home.htm

Singh, Mina D. (2004) Evaluation framework for nursing education programs: application of the CIPP model. *International Journal of Nursing Education Scholarship* 1(1), Article 13. [Online]: http://www.bepress.com/ijnes/vol1/iss1/art13

The Practice Quality Learning Evaluation Tool: http://www.pelqet.org.uk/index.php?pages_page_id=1000&dynamic_menus_page_id=1000

References

Attree, M. (2006) Evaluating healthcare education: issues and methods. *Nurse Education in Practice* 6(6), 332–8.

Bates, R. (2004) A critical analysis of evaluation practice: the Kirkpatrick model and the principle of beneficence. *Evaluation and Program Planning* 27, 341–47.

Cope, P., Cuthbertson, P. and Stoddart, B. (2000) Situated learning in the practice placement. *Journal of Advanced Nursing* 31(4), 850–6.

Cummins, F. (2006) Using auditing to enhance and improve practice. *Nursing and Residential Care* 8(1), 37–9.

Dean, J. (2000) The nature and purpose of evaluation. In Nicklin, P. and Kenworthy N. (eds), *Teaching and Assessing in Nursing Practice An Experiential Approach*, 3rd edn. London: Bailliere Tindall.

Department of Health (2001) *The Essence of Care Patient Focused Benchmarking for Healthcare Practitioners*. London: DoH.

Department of Health (2002) *Funding Learning and Development for the Healthcare Workforce*. London: DoH.

Department of Health (2003) *Essence of Care Patient Focussed Benchmarks for Clinical Governance*. London: DoH.

Donabedian, A. (1988) The quality of care. How can it be assessed? *American Journal of Public Health* 260(12), 1743.

Dunning, D., Johnson, K., Ehrlinger, J. and Kruger, J. (2003) Why people fail to recognise their own incompetence. *Current Directions in Psychological Science* 12(3), 83–7.

Garbett, R., Hardy, S., Manley, K., Titchen, A. and McCormack, B. (2007) Developing a qualitative approach to 360 Degree Feedback to aid understanding and development of clinical expertise. *Journal of Nursing Management* 15, 342–7.

General Social Care Council (GSCC) (2006) *Social Work Education in England: Listening, Learning and Shaping, The 2006 Social Work Education Quality Assurance Report.* London: General Social Care Council.

Gopee, N. (2008) *Mentoring and Supervision in Healthcare.* London: Sage Publications.

Gray, M. (2007) Learning and teaching. In Brooker, C. and Waugh, A. (eds), *Foundations of Nursing Practice Fundamentals of Holistic Care.* Edinburgh: Mosby Elsevier.

Health Professions Council (2007a) *Standards of Education and Training Guidance.* London: HPC.

Health Professions Council (2007b) *Fitness to Practice Annual Report 2007* London: HPC.

Jarvis, P. and Gibson, S. (1997) *The Teacher Practitioner and Mentor in Nursing, Midwifery, Health Visiting and the Social Services,* 2nd edn. Cheltenham: Stanley Thornes.

Langendyk, V. (2006) Not knowing that they do not know: self-assessment accuracy of third-year medical students. *Medical Education* 40, 173–9.

Mohanna, K., Wall, D. and Chambers, R. (2004) *Teaching Made Easy: A Manual for Health Professionals,* 2nd edn. Oxon: Radcliffe Medical Press Ltd.

Morris, J. (2007) Factors influencing the quality of student learning on practice placements. *Learning in Health and Social Care* 6(4), 213–19.

Neary, M. (2000) *Teaching, Assessing and Evaluation for Clinical Competence: A Practical Guide for Practitioners and Teachers.* Cheltenham: Nelson Thornes:

Nicklin, P. and Lankshear, A. (2000) The principles of assessment. In Nicklin, P. and Kenworthy, N. (eds), *Teaching and Assessing in Nursing Practice An Experiential Approach,* 3rd edn. London: Bailliere Tindall.

Nursing and Midwifery Council (2005) *Guidelines for Records and Record Keeping* London: NMC.

Nursing and Midwifery Council (2008) *Standards to Support Learning and Assessment in Practice, NMC standards for Mentors, Practice Teachers and Teachers.* London: NMC.

Phillips, T., Schostak, J and Tyler, J. (2000) *Practice and assessment in Nursing and Midwifery: Doing it for real (Researching Professional Education).* London: ENB.

Quality Assurance Agency for Higher Education (2005) *QAA Report on the Evaluation of Prototypes 2004–2005, Evaluation of the Prototypes for Ongoing Quality Monitoring, and Approval, Including the Evaluation of the Standards Template and Evidence Base.* Gloucester: QAA.

Quinn, F. and Hughes, S. (2007). Quinn's Principles and Practice of Nurse Education, 5th edn. Cheltenham: Nelson Thornes.

Rossi, P., Lipsey, M. and Freeman, H. (2004) *Evaluation a Systematic Approach,* 7th edn. Thousand Oaks, California: Sage Publications.

Singh, R. (2001) Peer evaluation: a process that could enhance the self-esteem and professional growth of teachers. *Education* 105(1), 73–5.

Stewart, J., O'Halloran, C., Barton, J., Singleton, S., Harrigan, P. and Spencer J. (2000) Clarifying the concepts of confidence and competence to produce appropriate self-evaluation measurement scales. *Medical Education* 34, 903–09.

Stufflebeam, D. (1971) The relevance of the CIPP evaluation model for educational accountability. *Journal of Research and Development in Education* 5(1), 1925.

Suls, J., Martin, R. and Wheeler, L. (2002) Social comparison: why, with whom, and with what effect? *Current Directions in Psychological Science* 11(5), 159.

Swalfield, S. and MacBeath, J. (2005) School self evaluation and the role of the critical friend. *Cambridge Journal of Education* 35(2), 239–52.

Vuorinen, R., Tarkka, M. and Meretoja, R. (2000) Peer evaluation in nurses' professional development: a pilot study to investigate the issues. *Journal of Clinical Nursing* 9, 273–81.

Ward, P. (1997) *360 Degree Feedback.* London: Institute of Personnel and Development.

12

Supervision and Support

Stephen Phillips, Claire Johnson, Vicky Kaye and Karen Adams

CHAPTER OBJECTIVES

Aim

To explore how clinical supervision can be used as a support mechanism in the practice setting.

Learning outcomes

- Appraise the role of clinical supervision in learning in practice.
- Analyse how feedback can be used to develop practice.
- Examine tools to facilitate student progression.

The role of clinical supervision in supporting Practice Teachers and students

Clinical supervision remains a cornerstone of professional practice within the arena of health and social care (Jones, 2003; Sellars, 2005; NMC, 2008). The pressures and constraints of public sector modernisation and re-organisation have impacted negatively on widespread and effective implementation, along with ongoing inconsistency and lack of commitment apparent within organisations (Edwards *et al.* 2005).

Research suggests that there are benefits to practitioners, organisations and service users when clinical supervision is effectively implemented (Arvidsson *et al.* 2001; Bowles and Young, 1999; Butterworth *et al.* 1997; Graham, 2000; Jones, 2003). However, disparity in the understanding and application of the concept coupled with lack of resources continue to undermine effective organisation (Cheater and Hale, 2001).

Butterworth (in Butterworth and Faugier, 1992, p. 12) defines clinical supervision as 'an exchange between practising professionals' and Bond and Holland (1998, p. 12) as 'regular protected time for facilitated in-depth reflection on clinical practice'. Defining clinical supervision as a structured framework for the application of critical reflection in practice relates closely to models of experiential learning (Boud *et al.* 1985) and can be usefully applied to the Practice Teacher both as a practitioner and in the role of educator and supporter of students. Similarly, as a modelling experience for students in practice, the value of developing skills in critical reflection and clinical supervision are evident as part of ongoing professional development.

The established purpose of clinical supervision also fits neatly with key aims for practice education that is; clinical governance, lifelong learning, practice development, facilitating best practice and support for the practitioner.

The expectation that high-quality clinical supervision will provide practitioners with the opportunity to access both support in the demanding field of health and social care practice (Hawkins and Shohet, 2006), and learning from critical debate about practice, has been long established (Butterworth and Faugier, 1992). Hawkins and Shohet (2006) highlight the importance of good supervision as a crucial habit we should establish early in our professional careers so that it becomes an integral part of our life at work. These key elements of clinical supervision are also strongly reflected

Table 12.1 Practice teaching and Proctor's model of supervision

Proctor's model of supervision	Examples of application to the Practice Teacher (PT) role with the student
Formative Educative Developmental Reflective	The PT will facilitate the student in reflecting on both observed practice (PT and others) and on their own (the student) practice during the placement. This may be immediate following the episode of care or at the end of the day. Positive and negative aspects of the experience will be explored and the PT may encourage the student to use a reflective model such as Gibb's (1988) to analyse their learning. The PT may give information and advice about the student's practice
Normative Competence Professional standards and ethics Protecting the public	The PT will explore with the student aspects of practice that present ethical dilemmas such as information sharing, consent and confidentiality. The PT may engage the student in considering legal requirements such as effective documentation and their duty of care.
Restorative Support De-briefing Emotional content of the work	The PT will allow the student to disclose their feelings about encounters in clinical practice such as anger and grief. The PT will affirm the student's worth and value and facilitates the student in coping with uncertainty and uncomfortable feelings.

in the principles of clinical governance with the emphasis on continuous improvement in the quality of care and the need to establish mechanisms to safeguard standards for patients and service users (Scally and Donaldson, 1998; DH, 1998).

The application of Brigid Proctor's three-function model of supervision embraces key areas of responsibility for the Practice Teacher (Proctor, 1986) Table 12.1.

Meeting the needs of Practice Teachers

Practice Teachers are practising professionals both as clinicians and as educators. It is therefore essential that clinical supervision caters to their needs as Practice Teachers in addition to the arena of practice. The Practice Teachers' clinical environment is the practicum of the student and the two aspects are inextricably linked (Twinn and Johnson 1998). Practice Teachers will need to access appropriate supervision that encompasses both dimensions. This may be specialist or non-specialist, group supervision or one to one (see Table 12.2).

Opportunities for multi-disciplinary supervision may be more accessible as organisational functions continue to embrace operational models that blur professional boundaries (Clouder and Sellars, 2004; DH, 2000, 2004; Davies *et al.* 2004; Launer, 2005). Multi-disciplinary education for clinical supervision can promote such opportunities as participants are able to make links with colleagues from different disciplines and agencies.

Table 12.2 Supervisor/participant criteria

Format	Same discipline background	Different discipline/has educational credentials	Peer supervision	Appointed facilitator	Rotating facilitator role	Supervisor support
Group	Colleagues from the same discipline background form group – across or beyond employing organisation	Colleagues from different discipline backgrounds form a supervision group	Peer supervision group – participants are of equal status/role avoids power imbalance	The group facilitator is appointed from either inside or outside the organisation- could be a consultant from another health organisation or from an educational establishment	The group participants take turns to act as facilitator	External facilitators usually have their own supervision. Rotating facilitation allows supervisors to obtain supervision from within the group
One to one	Access to recognised list/database of qualified supervisors to choose one from same discipline	Access to recognised supervisors from different discipline background	Co-supervision where two participants alternate sessions as supervisee and supervisor	–	–	Supervisors need to access their own supervision either as one-to-one or in a supervisors group

Source: Adapted from Houston, 1990.

Enhancing the student experience

Student practitioners can benefit from Practice Teachers modelling their educative role on that of clinical supervision (Saarikoski *et al.* 2006). Students will benefit from access to group and one-to-one experiences of learning that enable them to develop the skills required for critical reflection and clinical supervision. For example, challenging practice, giving and receiving feedback and being open to other perspectives. Challenge is a key responsibility in clinical supervision. It is a way of facilitating the development of self-awareness and identifying blocks to practice.

=== **ACTIVITY 12.1** ===

Arrange for yourself and your student to exchange feedback and provide challenge on a recent practice activity. This is best if the practice activity is relatively straightforward as more complex situations may prove too difficult to address within the context of this exercise. You could start by giving the student feedback on their role in the activity and then change roles so that the student then provides feedback on your observed input in the situation. Both of you should follow some simple rules during this process:

The environment should be 'safe' away from the busy office and the telephone.
Feedback should be specific not general.
Feedback should have immediacy not be saved up till the end of the discussion.
Presenting a range of options or choices when giving feedback opens up the opportunity for discussion.

Challenge should be positive.
Should be about the person's action not their personality.
May be about raising awareness of attitudes or behaviour.
You should be asking questions not making pronouncements.
Give each other time to think and respond.

(adapted from Bond and Holland, 1998)

It would be of great value to the student to observe or participate in supervision and most importantly, to have the opportunity to see in action how supervisory relationships are established. This process so eloquently detailed by Graham Sloan (Sloan, 2005) needs to be seen as skill- and knowledge-based in the same way as other 'clinical' skills and consequently requires the same level of teaching and learning opportunity.

Supervision is an established activity in social work. This is based on the principles outlined by Thomson (2006) related to ensuring that the learner is being supported in their practice whilst checking their ability to practice. Other aspects of this activity are concerned with providing a forum to discuss issues and an important function of the whole process is that the supervisee receives feedback on their ability to practice.

Using formative feedback to support student learning

Feedback is the central aspect of formative assessment as it is a key element in supporting learning and is significant in facilitating lifelong learning. According to Rushton (2005) the aim of the formative assessment process is to assist the development of the learner. This takes place through the provision of feedback about performance. A range of strategies can be utilised to support this.

One-to-one feedback

Feedback is about providing information about the existing gap between actual and desired level of performance (Rushton, 2005). It should also provide direction for improvement. Student involvement is seen as essential and a key strategy to facilitate this is through self-assessment mechanisms.

In order to provide effective support, formative assessment needs to be criterion referenced. Relevant reference points such as learning outcomes defined in learning contracts could all be utilised as a benchmark for measuring performance. In order to make the most of feedback, Rushton (2005) argues that this should be task centred. Practice Teachers are in an excellent position to offer such feedback as they are able to observe all aspects of clinical practice. Feedback should also be ongoing in order to maximise opportunities for knowledge and skills acquisition. Delaying positive feedback may lead to a loss of the motivational impact on learning (Stuart, 2003) and delaying negative feedback leads to a loss of opportunity to rectify problems and improve performance. Opportunities for feedback, for example, immediate feedback following a learning activity that a student has participated in, should be afforded wherever possible in addition to more structured and formal feedback. The practice portfolio is an important tool to support learning in practice and provide appropriate feedback as part of the process. Students can critically reflect on key aspects of their learning and experiences and record these in their practice portfolios. They are encouraged to consider these experiences in relation to course/module learning outcomes. This helps students to integrate theory and practice and can be assisted by using a structured reflective model such as John's (1995). Practice Teachers can therefore use the outcomes in the portfolio to offer formative feedback to support this process by directing and prompting students around key aspects of the experience.

Group feedback

Formative student-led case studies can be utilised in a group setting to support student learning. Students present a case scenario together with details of their role in the situation. This can then be followed by supportive feedback to each student from both Practice Teachers and peers. This can be effective in facilitating student learning as all participants are encouraged to think critically about the scenario and debate the practitioner's role. Disadvantages of this approach could include lack of support and commitment from peers and some students can become very anxious at the thought of such activity (Gopee, 2001). The emphasis must remain on mutual growth and support of the student. This approach also supports theory to practice link and can be facilitated by asking the students to think critically about how module and course learning outcomes relate.

=============================== **ACTIVITY 12.2** ===============================

Consider the use of group activities as a supportive mechanism in practice teaching in your area. How could the activities be facilitated? What are the advantages and challenges of giving and receiving feedback in a group situation? How would you identify that a student was feeling threatened by this approach?

Alternative feedback methods

Virtual learning environment

Most higher education establishments now have an established virtual learning environment such as 'Blackboard' or 'webCT' to support student learning. Within these virtual learning environments there are various asynchronous and synchronous tools such as discussion forums, chat rooms and electronic resources. This offers Practice Teachers an additional medium through which they can communicate with both students and academic staff. Denton *et al.* (2007) suggest that this medium facilitates both fair and balanced feedback as well as enabling feedback to be returned more quickly which may aid synthesis of information. Cramphorn (2004) (cited in Sharpe and Benfield, 2005), however, highlights the social and psychological barriers that can exist in relation to using electronic medium despite having adequate IT skills.

E-learning can also facilitate the development of supportive relationships between the students. This is of particular benefit to mature students who often work part-time and travel long distances to study their chosen course. This, of course, has IT training implications as a significant number of mature students (and Practice Teachers) have limited IT literacy. Fox and MacKeough (2003) point to some of these difficulties in engaging students in online activities. Academic staff and Practice Teachers therefore need to provide encouragement to students to access relevant training and participate in online activities. Linking online formative assessment tasks to summative assessment can provide some of the necessary impetus to encourage student contribution.

E-mail

Similar benefits and barriers exist in relation to the use of e-mail. The increased use and popularity of e-mail both in the workplace and at home suggest that it is an option that should not be ignored to improve the timeliness of feedback. It has the potential to improve contact and communication between the Practice Teacher, student and higher education institutes. This is crucial for motivation and improving student involvement and allows all concerned to communicate in a virtual group that does not take place in real time (Quinn and Hughes, 2007). Freedom from the constraints of location and time, potential for increased interaction, increased Internet experience and extended learning opportunities are benefits to this medium.

Written

A key characteristic of effective feedback is that it is provided soon after the observed behaviour (Parikh *et al.* 2001). It is therefore suggested that this method is utilised in conjunction with other strategies, such as one-to-one feedback, in order to ensure timeliness of feedback is not compromised. Written feedback provides an important record of student progression and achievement and contributes to the evidence required to confirm competency. It is therefore essential that it is legibly recorded and is criterion referenced, as discussed earlier.

=============== **ACTIVITY 12.3** ===============

Reflect on methods you have utilised to provide feedback to your students. Compare and contrast on their strengths and weaknesses.

Supporting Practice Teachers

Practice teachers have a dual role of teaching and practising as stated earlier. Whilst this can be a source of credibility with students it can also lead to situations where the practitioner has to manage the competing priorities of responding to clients and students. Practice teachers' support is available through a variety of mechanisms.

Intended learning outcomes are communicated to practice teachers through programme and module handbooks, practice documents, programme specifications and through university e-learning systems such as 'Blackboard'. Opportunities for clarification and discussion are afforded through study days and tripartite visits in the practice setting. The uses of virtual learning platforms also enable Practice Teachers to access information about activities that students are undertaking.

'The Standards for Practice Teachers of Nursing and Midwives' published in *Standards to Support Learning and Assessment in Practice* (NMC, 2008) determine a level of competence that Practice Teachers must be able to evidence in their professional portfolios in order to remain on a 'local' register of Practice Teachers held by the employer. Similarly other professions provided similar guidance (GMC, 2006; HPC, 2005). Practice Teachers are accountable for ensuring that their practice remains up to date and for seeking out appropriate professional development if necessary. This is formalised through annual appraisals and personal development planning. Higher education institutes and other organisations offer professional education to update Practice Teachers and ensure that they can maintain their competence. In addition to this higher education institutes can support placement providers in ensuring that Practice Teachers meet the requirements of their respective professional bodies.

Some higher education institutions have Practice Teacher panels, where a group of Practice Teachers come together to assess a cohort of student portfolios. This assists with moderation of practice learning and additionally is a good support mechanism for Practice Teachers (Shardlow and Doel, 1996). Practice Teachers can also provide effective support to one another through a range of peer support mechanisms. Experienced Practice Teachers are encouraged to provide preceptorship support to new Practice Teachers and this strategy has recently been formalised for nurses through the NMC circular 27/2007. Practice Teachers can also meet with their peers within or outside their employing organisation to share experiences and plan joint learning activities for their students.

Tools and strategies to support student learning

A key element in supporting students and Practice Teachers in the practice setting is the development of a tripartite arrangement as previously suggested. Tripartite structures were first seen in education through the Education Act 1944 (Batteson, 1999), where the education system was restructured to incorporate three levels of education: primary, secondary and higher.

Higher education institutes have developed this concept to incorporate a pre-planned meeting with the Practice Teacher, student and university lecturer (personal tutor), (Figure 12.1).

The purpose of this meeting is to discuss the students' progression, and to explore fully the relationship of integrating theory into the practice

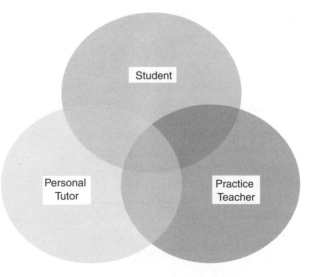

Figure 12.1 Tripartite relationship

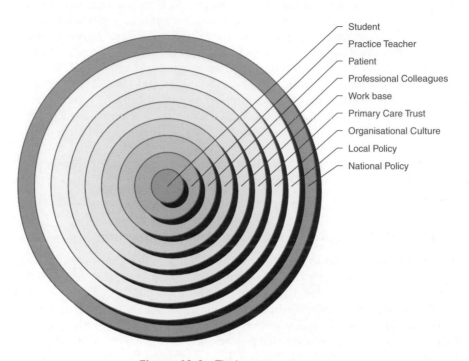

Student
Practice Teacher
Patient
Professional Colleagues
Work base
Primary Care Trust
Organisational Culture
Local Policy
National Policy

Figure 12.2   The learning environment

setting often utilising a practice portfolio. However, another option is to use a competency-based assessment tool to record a level of achievement. This meeting offers the opportunity to explore the experiences and challenges that both the student and Practice Teacher are exposed to.

In addition to the QAA Code, individual professional bodies will have their own codes/standards to support learning and assessment in practice; as referred to in Chapter 2. The learning environment can be seen as a multi-faceted concept, which in this situation can be viewed as the interaction between the student and Practice Teacher within the placement. Figure 12.2 demonstrates the complexity of the learning environment, all elements are all of equal importance to the students' experience.

In order to facilitate the learning of the individual student, learning contracts need to be developed. A learning contract can be seen as '... a means of reconciling the learning needs of the student and those of other interested parties such as educators and employers' (Quinn and Hughes, 2007, p. 30). Knowles (1990) identified key stages to the development of a learning contract (Figure 12.3). A learning contract is a valuable support mechanism within practice placements because it provides a formal, structured approach which enables the individual student to plan, develop and prioritise their own learning.

Stage 1: Diagnosis of learning needs
The learning needs are identified through the combination of the placement audit and the SWOT analysis.

Stage 2: Specifying the learning objectives
The learning objectives can be developed through specialist standards identified from specific professional bodies. Alternatively learning objectives can be developed from the learning needs identified through the SWOT analysis in stage one.

Stage 3: Specifying learning resources and strategies
This can be achieved through the development of individual 'action plans' based on each learning objective.

Stage 4: Specifying evidence of accomplishment
This can be demonstrated through the development of a professional portfolio. The evidence could be drawn from reflections 'in' and 'on' practice or presentation development and delivery.

Stage 5: Specifying how the evidence can be validated
This can be achieved through the use of formative and summative assessment by the practice teacher within the practice portfolio.

Stage 6: Reviewing the contract with consultants
This is undertaken within the tripartite structure where the learning contract is seen as one of the key tools for discussion.

Stage 7: Carrying out the contract
The student has the responsibility to carry out the specific learning contract and in partnership with the practice teacher review and amend accordingly.

Stage 8: Evaluating learning
The practice teacher has the responsibility to evaluate the students learning.
(Knowles, 1990)

Figure 12.3   Key Stages to the Development of a Learning Contract

The prime assessment tool for identifying learning needs within the learning contract is the development of a SWOT analysis, first identified in The Harvard Business School (Bryson, 1988). The SWOT analysis is the first stage of developing a learning contract as identified in Figure 12.3. The tool focuses on the strengths, weaknesses, opportunities and threats of a given situation. Practice Teachers are also encouraged to complete a SWOT analysis on the learning environment in order to recognise and develop the support mechanisms required for the students' learning experience. The following example (Figure 12.4) demonstrates the development of an identified learning need through the use of a SWOT analysis.

====== **ACTIVITY 12.4** ======

Reflect on the strategies described for student support. How do you assess your students' support needs? How could a SWOT analysis and learning contract be useful to you and your student in this process?

STRENGTHS	WEAKNESSES
Previous experience with basic Microsoft word, power-point and Internet searching. Willingness to learn. Being a student in a position to learn. Support from a practice teacher and team. A student on a course with a requirement to have access to local data.	Never utilised IT systems which access records and databases. Being a student not employed by the practice setting, hence, not being conversant with local IT systems and policies.
OPPORTUNITIES	THREATS
Training from practice teacher and team. Local 'in-house' training facilities on IT systems. Study time in practice. 'Cause for concern' policy in order to assist with negotiation of database access and training. Requirement to learn leadership and management skills as part of the course. Access to computer in the practice setting.	Time – the study day runs when the student is not available. Student not employed by placement organisation and hence not eligible for training or for passwords to access the databases.

Figure 12.4 SWOT Analysis (Information Technology Systems Within Placement)

Where students or Practice Teachers are experiencing difficulties which directly affects student learning, the support mechanisms developed should be seen as a tool to identify concerns in the learning process. Any actions can then be identified and formalised to ensure that the student is fully supported throughout the process. An example of this structure can be seen in the development of a 'cause for concern' process (Figure 12.5). This can be seen as a fair and equitable process which identifies the pertinent issues and a joint action plan can be developed to ensure resolution of the issue. Chapter 10 provides further discussion on managing challenging situations.

ACTIVITY 12.5

Consider the 'cause for concern' flow chart (Figure 12.5).
Think of an issue that has affected student learning. Consider the flow chart and work through the process. Reflect on the appropriateness of this tool and how it could be used as a supportive mechanism in your area.

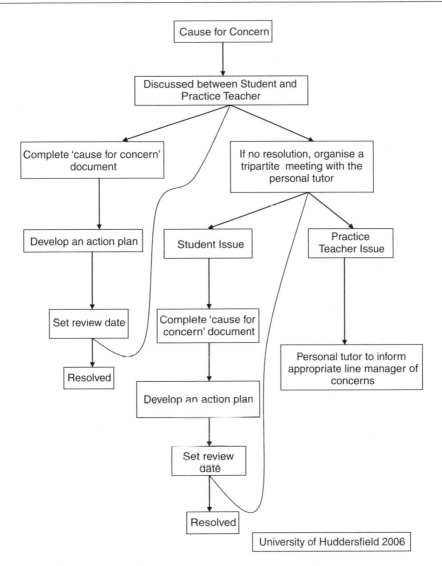

Figure 12.5 Flow chart demonstrating the 'cause for concern' process

Conclusion

In order to gain the long-term benefits of effective clinical supervision it is essential that a critical mass of practitioners equipped with the knowledge and skills to engage in clinical supervision are established. Practice Teachers can play a vital role in facilitating the development of the essential skills and knowledge for clinical supervision by engaging students in active supervision experience during practice placement experience. As clinical leaders in practice, Practice Teachers can also act as advocates for effective supervision by exerting their collective influence on peers, educators and employing organisations.

Formative feedback is a key method for supporting learning, which is useful to both the student and Practice Teacher in the progression of learning. Feedback is essential and can be completed utilising a variety of methods including the use of modern technologies.

The development of tripartite arrangements is a method of enhancing the student learning experience. Supporting Practice Teachers in the development of the learning environment, and developing their skills in supervision and feedback, is also key to educational excellence. Tools such as the SWOT analysis play a vital role in the understanding and appreciation of the students' needs. The 'cause for concern' process is an example demonstrating a collaborative approach to problem solving.

Resources

Driscoll, J. (2000) *Practising Clinical Supervision A Reflective Approach.* London: Harcourt Publications.

Hawkins, P. and Shoet, R. (2000) *Supervision in the Helping Professions.* Buckingham: Open University Press.

Heron, J. (1999) *The Complete Facilitator's Handbook.* London: Kogan Page.

Johns, C. (2000) *Becoming a Reflective Practitioner. A Reflective and Holistic Approach to Clinical Nursing, Practice Development and Clinical Supervision.* Cambridge: Blackwell Science.

Rolfe, G., Freshwater, D., and Jasper, M. (2001) *Critical Reflection For Nursing And The Helping Professions: A User's Guide.* Basingstoke: Palgrave.

Winstanley, J. and White, E. (2003) Clinical supervision: models, measures and best practice. *Nurse Researcher* 10 (4), 8–38.

References

Arvidsson, B., Lofgren, H. and Fridlund, B. (2001) Psychiatric nurses conceptions of how a group supervision programme in nursing care influences their professional competence: a 4-year follow up study. *Journal of Nursing Management* 9, 161–71.

Batteson, C.H. (1999) The 1944 education act reconsidered.

Educational Review, 51(1), 5–15.

Bond, M. and Holland, S. (1998) *Skills of Clinical Supervision for Nurses.* Buckingham: Open University Press.

Boud, D., Keogh, R. and Walker, D. (eds) (1985) *Reflection: Turning Experience Into Learning.* London: Kogan Paul.

Bowles, N. and Young, C. (1999) An evaluative study of clinical supervision based on proctor's three function interactive model. *Journal of Advanced Nursing* 30(4) 958–64.

Bryson, J.M. (1988) *Strategic Planning for Public and Nonprofit Organisations.* San Francisco: Jossey-Bass.

Butterworth, T., White, E., Jeacock, J., Clements, A. and Bishop, V. (1997) *It is Good to Talk.* Manchester: University of Manchester: School of Nursing, Midwifery and Health Visiting.

Butterworth, T. and Faugier, J. (1992) *Clinical Supervision and Mentorship in Nursing.* London: Chapman and Hall.

Cheater, F.M. and Hale, C. (2001) An evaluation of a local clinical supervision scheme for practice nurses. *Journal of Clinical Nursing* 10, 119–31.

Clouder, L. and Sellars, J. (2004) Reflective practice and clinical supervision: an interprofessional perspective. *Journal of Advanced Nursing* 46(3), 262–9.

Davies, E.J., Tennant, A., Ferguson, E. and Jones, L.F. (2004) Developing models and a framework for multi-professional clinical supervision. *British Journal of Forensic Practice* 6(3), 36–42.

Denton, P., Madden, J., Roberts, M. and Rowe, P. (2007) Students' response to traditional and computer assisted formative feedback: a comparative case study. *British Journal of Educational Technology*, Online Early Articles Published article [Online]: 16-Aug-2007 doi: 10.1111/j.1467–8535.2007.00745.x

Department for Education and Skills (2003) *Widening Participation in Higher Education.* Cheshire: DfES.

Department of Health (1998) *A First Class Service: Quality in the New NHS.* London: DH.

Edwards, D., Cooper, L., Burnard, P., Hannigan, B., Adams, J., Fothegill, A. and Coyle, D. (2005) Factors influencing the effectiveness of clinical supervision. *Journal of Psychiatric and Mental Health Nursing* 12, 405–14.

Fox, S. and MacKeogh, K. (2003) Can eLearning promote higher-order learning without tutor overload? *Open Learning: The Journal of Open and Distance Learning* 18(2), 12–34.

General Medical Council (2006) *Good Medical Practice.* London: General Medical Council.

Gibbs, G. (1988) *Learning by Doing: A Guide to Teaching and Learning Methods.* Oxford: Oxford Polytechnic.

Gopee, N. (2001) The Role of Peer Assessment and Peer Review in Nursing *British Journal of Nursing* 9(11), 724–729.

Graham, I.W. (2000) Reflective practice and its role in mental health nurses' practice development: a year long study. *Journal of Psychiatric and Mental Health Nursing* 7, 109–17.

Hawkins, P. and Shohet, R. (2006) *Supervision in the Helping Professions.* London: Kogan Page.

Health Professions Council (2005) Continuing Professional Development – Key Decisions. London: Health professions Council.

Houston, G. (1990) Supervision and Counselling. London: The Rochester Foundation.

Johns, C. (1995) Framing learning through reflection within carper's fundamental ways of knowing in nursing. *Journal of Advanced Nursing* 22, 226–34.

Jones, A. (2003) Some benefits experienced by hospice nurses from group clinical supervision. *European Journal of Cancer Care* 12, 224–32.

Knowles, M. (1990) *The Adult Learner: A Neglected Species*, 4th edn. Houston: Gulf Publishing.

Launer, J. (2005) Reflective Practice and Clinical Supervision: demonstrating clinical supervision to GP educators. *Work based Learning in Primary Care* 3, 159–161.

Nursing Midwifery Council (2001) *Standards for Specialist Education and Practice.* London: NMC.

Nursing and Midwifery Council (2006) *Standards to Support Learning and Assessment in Practice: NMC Standards for Mentors, Practice Teachers and Teachers.* London: NMC.

Nursing and Midwifery Council (2007) *Sign off Status and Preceptorship for Practice Teacher Students, Circular 27/2007.* London: NMC.

Parikh, A., McReelis, K. and Hodges, B. (2001) Student feedback in problem based learning: a survey of 103 final year students across five Ontario medical schools. *Medical Education* 35(7), 632–6.

Proctor, B. (1986) Supervision: a cooperative exercise in accountability. In Marken, M., and Payne, M. (eds), *Enabling and Ensuring.* Leicester: Leicester Youth Bureau and Training in Community Work.

Quality Assurance Agency (2001) *Code of Practice for the Assurance of Academic Quality and Standards in Higher Education: Section 9: Placement Learning.* [Online]. <http://www.qaa.ac.uk/academicinfrastructure/codeOfPractice/section9/default.asp> (accessed 21 February 2007).

Quinn, F. and Hughes, S. (2007) Quinn's Principles and Practice of Nurse Education, 5th edn. Cheltenham: Nelson Thornes Publishers.

Rushton, A. (2005) Formative assessment: a key to deep learning? *Medical Teacher* 27(6), 509–13.

Saariskoski, M., Warne, T., Aunio, R. and Leino-Kilpi, H. (2006) Group supervision in facilitating learning and teaching in mental health clinical placements: a case example of one student group. *Issues in Mental Health Nursing* 27(3), 273–85.

Scally, G. and Donaldson, L.J. (1998) The NHS's 50th Anniversary. Looking Forward. Clinical Governance and the Drive for a Quality Improvement in the New NHS in England. [Online] http://www.bmj.com/cgi/content/full/317/7150/61 (accessed 9 January 2008).

Sellars, J. (2005) Learning from contemporary practice: an exploration of clinical supervision in physiotherapy. *Learning in Health and Social Care* 3(2), 64–82.

Shardlow, S. and Doel, M. (1996) *Practice Learning and Teaching*. Basingstoke: Macmillan.

Sharpe, R. and Benfield, G. (2005) The student experience of e-learning in higher education. *Brookes eJournal of Learning and Teaching* 1(3).

Sloan, G. (2005) Clinical supervision: beginning the supervisory relationship. *British Journal of Nursing* 14(17), 918–23.

Stuart, C. (2003) *Assessment Supervision and Support in Clinical Practice*. Edinburgh: Elsevier Science Ltd.

Thompson, N. (2006) *Promoting Workplace Learning*. Bristol: The Policy Press.

Twinn, S. and Johnson, C. (1998) in Butterworth, T., Faugier, J., and Burnard, P. (eds) *Clinical Supervision and Mentorship in Nursing*. Cheltenham: Stanley Thornes Ltd.

University of Huddersfield (2006) *BSc(Hons)/MSc Community Nursing Practice Student Handbook*. Huddersfield: University of Huddersfield.

The Expert Practitioner

Heather McAskill

CHAPTER OBJECTIVES

Aim

To explore the notion of the Practice Teacher as the expert practitioner.

Learning outcomes

- Analyse professionalism within the role of the Practice Teacher.
- Evaluate the concept of expert practice as a Practice Teacher.
- Appraise the role of the Practice Teacher in practice and curriculum development.
- Examine the value of training needs analysis.

It is often assumed that because one has a professional qualification one is an expert. In reality the role of the Practice Teacher is complex. To be able to examine a student's practice the Practice Teacher must first be able to examine his or her own. This can be extremely challenging unless they are confident of their abilities and the evidence base for their own work, and are able to use reflection in their work. In essence a Practice Teacher must be an expert practitioner (Benner, 1984).

Professionalism

Prior to discussing the concept of 'expert practitioner' as a Practice Teacher of health professionals, it is useful to consider the term 'profession'. Styles (2005) lists the following characteristics of a true profession: higher education; distinct service or practice; evidence-based knowledge; autonomy; code of ethics and a regulatory body. Nursing like many other occupation has been engaged in the process of profession building as its education has moved into higher education institutes and aims for a graduate profession (Allen, 2007). The United Kingdom Standard Occupational Classification classifies nurses and the allied health professionals in the third major occupational group entitled 'associate, professional and technical occupations' whereas medical practitioners and pharmacists are classified in the second major occupational group entitled 'professional occupations' (National Statistics, 2000). Interestingly, teachers of primary, secondary and tertiary education are considered in group two. In relation to the education of health professionals, those who support education in the clinical area are still considered in group three, whereas health professionals who move into higher education within a teaching role are considered a 'professional' using this classification and have moved into the second group. The main argument for this appears to be that as a health professional within higher education not only is subject expertise required but also educational expertise to be regarded as a true professional (Kenny, 2004; NMC, 2008; Watts, 2000). This does help to explain the current emphasis on the accreditation of teaching in higher education (NMC, 2008). However, this classification of professions appears to be part of the UK culture and is very hierarchical (Watson, 2000). What is more important within the role of the Practice Teacher is the term 'professionalism'.

The Royal College of Nursing (2003) distinguished between professional nursing and nursing undertaken by other unqualified people to clarify professionalism. The difference lies in the clinical judgement processes, underpinning knowledge, personal accountability and the professional regulation; all of which are essential elements of clinical practice. This distinction could be applied to other health professions and also supports Eraut's (1994) core concepts of professionalism: specialist knowledge base, autonomy and service. The concept that a professional has a specialist knowledge base is the key to the ideology of professionalism. In terms of higher education it is this knowledge that underpins professional judgement and decisions in practice (Watts, 2000). Considering the second concept of professionalism, having high levels of professional autonomy as a Practice Teacher is essential, despite the increasing monitoring and quality processes within higher education and clinical practice which at times can be restraining. The autonomous practitioner needs to be fully aware of the responsibilities inherent within that autonomy and consider ethical and professional requirements. The authority to take decisions, actions and risks is viewed as a key component of expertise. Eraut's (1994) final concept is service, which is the relationship you may have with your students. This relationship was traditionally seen as an unequal power relationship (Watts, 2000), and still is the case in some undergraduate education. However, as Eraut (1994) notes, the traditional notion of the professional being in a dominant position of power is changing to a facilitative relationship. It is clear that in considering the characteristics of professionalism, Practice Teachers demonstrate many of them. They need to show an awareness of the salient issues and be 'experts' in their field.

Expert practice

Some of the readers of this chapter may presently consider themselves to be experts in their field of practice. Others may be reluctant to adopt such a title. It may be that in some situations practitioners feel confident of their abilities, whilst in others there could be doubts.

ACTIVITY 13.1

Make notes about a situation in which you feel that you demonstrated your own expertise. Include the following observations:

■ What makes your input that of an expert?

■ What factors did you consider at the time?

■ How did you develop expertise?

The definition of 'expert practice' within professional practice is open to debate; for some it is an objective concept, others regard it as an intuition underpinned by deep understanding and experience (Benner, 1984; Dreyfus, 1982). The Dreyfus model (Dreyfus, 1982; Dreyfus and Dreyfus, 1986) consists of five stages of progress: novice, advanced beginner, competent, proficient and expert. The focus of this model is that individuals can proceed from being novices where they are governed by rules to help them carry out tasks to experts which rely on a deep tacit knowledge to act intuitively in a given situation.

Benner (1984) in her seminal work applied this model to explore the notion of intuition in expert practice within nursing practice and challenged the fact that 'skill is the mere application of knowledge'. In Benner's description of each stage there is a significant difference between competent and expert, the competent practitioner consistently uses an analytical framework for conscious and deliberate planning, whereas 'expert' is defined as someone who no longer practices by formally analysing every decision, but practices intuitively based on the experience of having met the situation before. Other professions have examined this work and have recognised similar complexities in their own practice.

Manley and McCormack (1997) critically analysed the literature relating to nursing practice expertise and identified five attributes characterising practice:

1. Holistic practice knowledge

2. Knowing the patient

3. Saliency

4. Moral agency

5. Skilled know-how

These attributes help to define expertise within practice. Hardy *et al.* (2006) undertook a study of a variety of nurses throughout the United Kingdom and recognised the importance of expertise in health care. They provided a case study of an acute situation to demonstrate this. Saliency can be seen in the practitioner identifying the problem from non-verbal clues. Skilled know-how was evident by the response rate. Knowing the patient and moral agency were demonstrated in the rapport building with the patient and carer and holistic practice knowledge can be seen in the involvement of all relevant professionals. Manley *et al.*'s study (2005) added to the current understanding of what practice expertise involves and identified two additional attributes. First, the concept that expert practitioners are risk takers in that they are prepared to take action outside conventional practice and second that they act as catalysts for change (Hardy *et al.* 2006).

It could be suggested that these attributes could be transferable to other professional roles and also to your role as a Practice Teacher with the adoption of attribute one to encompass specialist knowledge:

1. Specialist knowledge

2. Knowing the student

3. Saliency

4. Moral agency

5. Skilled know-how

6. Risk taker

7. Change catalyst

Manley and McCormack (1997) also identified a range of enabling factors for the development of expertise which can be considered in all areas of professional practice:

1. Reflectivity

2. Organisation

3. Interpersonal relationships

4. Autonomy and authority

5. Recognition by others

Reflexivity refers 'to the way in which all accounts of social settings – descriptions, analyses, criticisms – and the social settings occasioning them, are mutually interdependent' (Cohen *et al.* 2000, p. 25). In other words, it is not a single event but a process. Reflection is discussed more fully in a separate chapter, however in this context it is clear that reflection is important not only to expose expertise but also to encourage practitioners to analyse and synthesise their practice in a purposeful way (Hardy *et al.* 2006).

Organisation suggests that expert practice requires the ability to prioritise and delegate amongst and across teams. Likewise developing and maintaining effective interpersonal relationships is a key requisite of expert practice. Baumann (2006) suggests that interpersonal skills should be an attribute of clinical expertise rather than an enabling factor. However, it is clear that expertise is a complex process with many overlapping factors. It is apparent that there are interrelationships between the attributes and enabling factors and as long as they are all considered it is immaterial.

Autonomy and authority is the fourth enabling factor identified and is a key attribute of expert practice and is embedded within higher degrees (QAA, 2001; Department of Health, 2004; SCQF, 2003). Making difficult decisions and being accountable for the consequences is a key component of expertise. Finally, recognition by others is the last enabling factor of expertise.

Eraut and Du Boulay (2000) in their review of the literature emphasised that it is the process that experts use their knowledge, as much as the quantity of the knowledge, which defines expertise. Clinical reasoning is optimised in the expert's area of practice, and rather than be a hypothetico-deductive approach, differs from situation to situation. Theories of expertise developed in different contexts, using different research methodologies may focus on different characteristics, but do not greatly differ in their conclusions (Eraut and du Boulay, 2000). In fact you can argue that many of the concepts overlap with professionalism. Understanding expertise is important for self-development, sharing knowledge with others and supporting student's learning.

ACTIVITY 13.2

Now consider the above theories in relation to your dual role as a clinical practitioner and a Practice Teacher. Consider the knowledge, skills and attributes you require in both roles and consider where you would be placed in Benner's continuum (Figure 13.1).

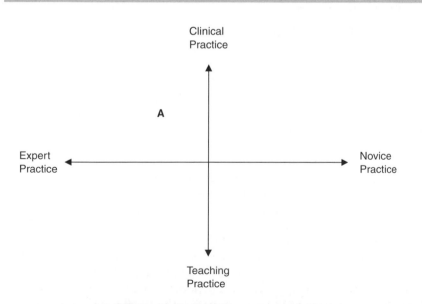

Figure 13.1 The novice to expert continuum

Most Practice Teachers within their field of expertise will operate during the majority of the time in position A. However, different situations will depend on where they sit in that position and they will fluctuate across the continuum. For example, if a practitioner takes on a new role as a non-medical prescriber they may see themselves as a novice adhering rigidly to guidelines; however, transferable knowledge and skills can be employed to assist in the journey towards 'expert' practice. As indicated previously expert practice involves being a catalyst of change and increasingly the practitioner may have to operate out with zone A. This involves being responsible for their own practice, where intuition, judgement and taking risks become important. Specialist knowledge is still essential but is insufficient on its own (Benner, 1984; Hardy *et al.* 2006; Stephenson, 1998).

In this conceptualisation it could be argued that it is difficult to achieve dual expertise. There is an assumption that if one is an 'expert' in clinical practice one will automatically be 'expert' in transmitting that knowledge to novices (Little and Milliken, 2007). Considering Benner's classification of 'expert' perhaps it is more realistic to strive for 'competence' in the role of a Practice Teacher. Similarly, it may be more achievable for academic staff within higher education institutions to aim for 'expert' within education and 'competence' in clinical practice, as maintaining expertise in clinical practice with the relevant setting is challenging. This is where professional standards in the role of a Practice Teacher can support practice (NMC, 2008). Effective performance draws on all elements of expertise and in the role of a Practice Teacher this will be apparent in many areas and in particular as a bridge between the theory–practice gap. One way of addressing this is considering the input that Practice Teachers can make within curriculum development.

Curriculum development

Curriculum development is a complex process involving more than just educational considerations (Goldenberg *et al.* 2004). It is a combination of theory and practice and requires careful facilitation to promote integration. There are many frameworks available to support this process (Armitage *et al.* 1999; CELT, 2002; Douglis, 1994; Humphreys, 1994; Nicklin and Kenworthy, 2000; Quinn and Hughes, 2007). Some of the models only focus on curriculum design that is the structure, content and process, rather than the broader concept of curriculum development which involves exploratory stage, design, implementation and monitoring and review (Quinn and Hughes, 2007). However, they all attempt to provide educational links between the objectives, course content, teaching and learning methods and the assessment of learning while considering the students' characteristics and multiple learning styles. As it is an ongoing process the linear models (Armitage *et al.* 1999; Humphreys, 1994) are not always as useful as the flow diagram (CELT, 2002). Douglis's cylindrical model (1994) does not consider all the elements within the linear models and the flow diagram, but outlines components to be considered for an integrated instructional design and provides the framework for a blended approach to learning. Figure 13.2 conceptualises the integration of these models

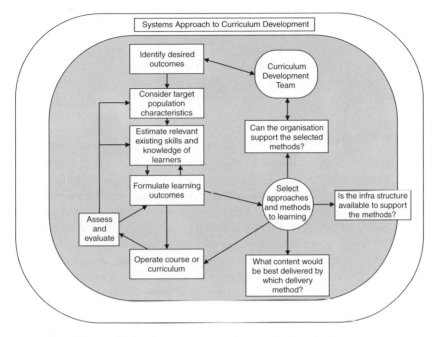

Figure 13.2 A systems approach to curriculum development

and provides a systems approach to curriculum development demonstrating the interrelationships between the elements and how changes in one element can have an impact on others.

The identification of the desired outcomes is a key stage in starting the process. This stage requires an analysis of the perceived need, considering educational institution's requirements, professional regulations and the needs of service. Depending on this information will depend on the members of the curriculum development team. A development team consisting of relevant academic staff from the university, users, and key people from clinical practice who consider clinical demands, staffing levels, the geographic spread of potential students, the cost of releasing staff from the workplace and the relevant national guidelines is vital to successful curriculum design. This is where practitioners such as Practice Teachers are essential in the process, professional practice is continually evolving and it is essential that curriculum is relevant to the needs of practice.

ACTIVITY 13.3

Consider this systems approach to course development. What is your role as a Practice Teacher within each of the elements of the model?

Traditionally curriculum development has been dominated by educational institutions but in order to meet the needs of service providers and provide quality practice education a more collaborative team approach is required (Glen and

Parker, 2003; Quinn and Hughes, 2007). Encouraging Practice Teachers to engage in curriculum development will help to facilitate the process. It is clear that as well as subject expertise Practice Teachers have knowledge of the target group population, the main clinical areas in which they will work allowing the team to estimate the relevant existing skills and knowledge of the students to aid the development of the curriculum.

Practice development

Health and social care provision continues to be shaped by politics, which requires effective leaders to translate this policy in a meaningful way to influence practice and support professional development. As a Practice Teacher and an 'expert' in one's field a commitment to lead and contribute to practice developments to meet the needs of practice is required (DoH, 2004). Prior to considering the Practice Teacher's role within practice development it is useful to define the term as there is often misunderstanding about the term 'practice development'.

The definition of practice itself is clear, however there appears to be contradictions in what is meant by development (Griffiths, 2003; McCormack *et al.* 2006). Within NHS Research and Development strategies, development is more often regarded as applied research (DoH, 2006). It can be argued that developing practice encompasses more than implementing research findings and in some areas of practice there is little research available to inform practice. A broader definition of practice development is a collection of processes which support individuals, teams and organisations to improve health care by sharing examples of good practice to the benefit of the public and the organisation (NHS Quality Improvement Scotland, 2007; Sale, 2005). Unsworth (2000) suggests that practice development should always be patient focused and involves:

- Introduction of new ways of working, which leads to a measurable improvement to the care/service to the patient.

- Changes that occur as a response to a patient problem.

- Changes that lead to the development of effective services.

- The maintenance or development of the professional or organisation.

This indicates that it is a continuous and incremental process. Practice development is therefore an essential element of clinical governance, a systematic approach to managing quality assurance improvement (Sale, 2005). All practitioners have a role within practice development and should be enabled to do so. It should be planned and integral to the strategic direction of the service or it will be difficult to sustain (Gerrish and Ferguson, 2000).

Gerrish *et al.* (2003) identify five principles that can be used to guide practice development:

- Providing a client-orientated service
- Team working

- Working collaboratively with the local community and other agencies

- Enabling practitioners to realise their potential

- Adopting a systematic approach to practice development

There is a lack of clarity regarding relevant methodologies within practice development, but this has not prevented practice development in recent years. No one methodological perspective can address all practice development functions. However, all should contain evidence of participatory, inclusive and collaborative methodology (McCormack *et al.* 2006). What is vital in the process is the engagement of relevant practitioners to deliver practice development. As an expert in their field the Practice Teacher is key to influence and manage new practice developments and use these to facilitate student's learning.

ACTIVITY 13.4

Reflect on your experience of practice development within your profession and consider the following:

- Which of these principles are evident in your practice?
- How did you measure the outcomes?
- What factors impacted on the outcomes?
- How does practice development contribute to a learning culture?

Training needs analysis

A Practice Teacher who promotes the concepts of adult learning needs to embrace this philosophy and demonstrate his/her competence as a teacher. Learning to assess and reassess competence to identify continuing professional development needs becomes increasingly complex as one progresses through one's professional career (Eraut and du Boulay, 2000). In fact, continuing professional development should be viewed as a continuum throughout practice, from 'novice to expert' (Gould *et al.* 2007). Training needs analysis tools are valuable in identifying training and development needs of practitioners and are regarded as a way of improving service delivery (Gould *et al.* 2004). Many of the tools referred to throughout this book that can be used with students, will be valuable resources when considering the Practice Teacher's needs. However, in order for Practice Teachers to meet their professional requirements they may wish to consider something more specific to their own profession.

For example, the General Medical Council (GMC, 2006) provides the principles and values that medical professionalism is based on. This could be developed into a training needs analysis tool when considering the requirements for teaching, training, appraising and assessing as illustrated below (Table 13.1). In order to complete such a tool the Practice Teacher needs to reflect on his/her role as a Practice Teacher, make a self-assessment of one's knowledge and skills, consider any supporting evidence and then identify any areas where one would benefit from further training, education and development. Similarly, the Nursing and Midwifery Council (NMC, 2008) *Standards to Support Learning and Assessment in Practice: NMC Standards for Mentors, Practice Teachers and Teachers* can be used to develop a Practice Teacher training needs analysis tool using the NMC outcomes (Table 13.2).

Enlisting the help of other people to obtain a more objective view of learning needs can also be useful. After undertaking such an analysis this information can be developed into a personal development plan to identify how any learning deficits will be addressed, and the evidence collated into a portfolio for future reference. This can be integrated within an existing professional portfolio (GMC, 2006; HPC, 2005; NMC, 2004) or a portfolio specific to the role of a Practice Teacher.

Table 13.1 Practice Teacher training needs analysis tool using GMC principles and values

Principles and values	Level of confidence			Evidence
	1	2	3	
Teaching and training, appraising and assessing				
Teaching, training, appraising and assessing doctors and students are important for the care of patients now and in the future. You should be willing to contribute to these activities.				
If you are involved in teaching you must develop the skills, attitudes and practices of a competent teacher.				
You must make sure that all staff for whom you are responsible, including locums and students, are properly supervised.				
You must be honest and objective when appraising or assessing the performance of colleagues, including locums and students. Patients will be put at risk if you describe as competent someone who has not reached or maintained a satisfactory standard of practice.				
You must provide only honest, justifiable and accurate comments when giving references for, or writing reports about, colleagues. When providing references you must do so promptly and include all information that is relevant to your colleague's competence, performance or conduct.				

1. I require training and development in most or all of this area.
2. I require training and development in some aspects of this area.
3. I am confident I already do this competently.

Table 13.2 Practice Teacher training needs analysis tool using NMC outcomes

Outcome	Level of confidence			Evidence
	1	2	3	
Establishing effective working relationships				
Have effective professional and inter-professional working relationships to support learning for entry to the register and education at a level beyond initial registration.				
Be able to support students moving into specific areas of practice or a level of practice beyond initial registration, identifying their individual needs in moving to a different level of practice.				
Support mentors and other professionals in their roles to support learning across practice and academic learning environments.				

1. I require training and development in most or all of this area.
2. I require training and development in some aspects of this area.
3. I am confident I already do this competently.

=========================== **ACTIVITY 13.5** ===========================

Review your professional portfolio and consider the following:

▦ Does your portfolio present an accurate representation of your practice?
▦ What specific examples of evidence from your experience as a Practice Teacher would you include in your portfolio?
▦ Is the structure of your portfolio logical?
▦ Have you included a relevant cross-referencing grid or matrix to any competencies?
▦ Have you included your personal development plan?
▦ Could you portfolio be developed to an e-portfolio?

The value of portfolios in student learning has been discussed throughout this book and the principles are the same for both the student and the Practice Teacher. It is a visual representation for demonstrating expertise, and needs to involve critical reflection and provide evidence of continuing professional development and lifelong learning, and competence as a Practice Teacher (McCready, 2007).

Conclusion

This chapter has explored the complexities of the concept of the expert practitioner, considering professionalism and some selected theories relating to expert practice within your role as a Practice Teacher. Determining expertise is difficult, but it is important to understand it to facilitate student learning. This concept is examined further in the Practice Teacher's as a subject expert, within a systems approach to curriculum development. Practice development is briefly discussed, acknowledging there is a lack of clarity in some of the methodologies; however, this should not prevent practitioners from advancing practice. Finally, training needs analysis tools are considered to identify professional development needs to maintain competence as a Practice Teacher and move along the continuum to 'expert' (Benner, 1984).

Resources

Developing Change Management Skills. A Resource for Health Care Professionals and Managers. [Online] http://www.sdo.lshtm.ac.uk/publications.htm
Critical Appraisal Skills Programme. [Online] http://www.phru.org.uk/~casp/index.htm
E-Portfolios. [Online] http://www.eportfolios.ac.uk/
Joseph Rowntree Foundation. [Online] http://www.jrf.org.uk/research-and-policy/
NHS Leadership Qualities Framework. [Online] http://www.nhsleadershipqualities.nhs.uk/
Practice-based Learning. [Online] http://www.practicebasedlearning.org/home.htm

References

Allen, D. (2007) What do you do at Work? Profession building and doing nursing. International Nursing Review 54(1), 41–8.
Armitage, A., Bryant, R., Dunnill, R., Hammersley, M., Hayes, D., Hudson, A. and Lawes, S. (1999) Teaching and Training in Post-compulsory Education. Buckingham: Open University Press.
Baumann, S. (2006) What does expert nursing practice mean? Nursing Science Quarterly 19, 259–60.
Benner, P. (1984) Novice to Expert: Excellence and Power: Clinical Nursing Practice. Menlo Park CA: Addison Wesley.
Centre for the Enhancement of Learning and Teaching (2002) Principles of Teaching, Learning and Assessment. Aberdeen: The Robert Gordon University.
Cohen, L., Lawrence, M. and Morrison, K. (2000) Research Methods in Education, 5th edn. London: Routledge Falmer.
Department of Health (2004) The NHS Knowledge and Skills Framework and the Development Review Process. London: DH.
Department of Health (2006) Best Research for Best Health: A New National Health Strategy. London: DH.
Douglis, F. (1994) Blended Learning: Choosing the Right Blend. [Online] http://coe.sdsu.edu/eet/articles/blendlearning/index.htm (accessed 3 December 2007).
Dreyfus, H. and Dreyfus, S. (1985) Mind Over Machine. New York: Macmillan.
Dreyfus, S. (1982) Formal models human situational understanding: inherent limitations on the modelling of business expertise. Office: Technology and People 1, 133–65.
Eraut, M. (1994) Developing Professional Knowledge and Competence. London: Falmer Press.
Eraut, M. and du Boulay, B. (2000) Developing the Attributes of Medical Professional Judgement and Competence. [Online] http://www.cogs.susx.ac.uk/users/bend/doh (accessed 11 October 2007).
General Medical Council (2006) Good Medical Practice. London: General Medical Council.
Gerrish, K. and Ferguson, A. (2000) Nursing development units: factors influencing their progress. British Journal of Nursing 9(10), 626–30.

Gerrish, K., Dorsman, J., Whitfiled, N. and Mischenko, J. (2003) Nursing development units: a model for promoting practice development in primary care. In Bryar, R. and Griffiths, J. (eds), Practice Development in Community Nursing. London: Arnold.

Glen, S. and Parker, P. (2003) Supporting Learning in Nursing Practice: A Guide for Practitioners. Basingstoke: Palgrave Macmillan.

Goldenberg, D., Andrusyszyn, M. and Iwasiw, C. (2004) A facilitative approach to learning about curriculum development. Journal of Nursing Education 43(1), 31–5.

Gould, D., Kelly, D. and White, I. (2004) Training-needs analysis: an evaluation framework. Nursing Standard 18(20), 33–6.

Gould, D., Drey, N. and Berridge, E. (2007) Nurses' experiences of continuing professional development. Nurse Education Today 27, 602–09.

Griffiths, J. (2003) Practice development: defining the terms. In Bryar, R. and Griffiths, J. Practice Development in Community Nursing. London: Arnold.

Hardy, S., Titchen, A., Manley, K. and McCormack, B. (2006) Re-defining nursing expertise in the united kingdom. Nursing Science Quarterly 19(3), 260–4.

Health Professions Council (2005) Continuing Professional Development – Key Decisions. London: Health Professions Council.

Humphreys, J. (1994) cited in Quinn, F. (2001) Quinn's Principles and Practice of Nurse Education 4th edn. Salisbury: Stanley Thornes.

Kenny, G. (2004) The origins of current nurse education policy and its implications for nurse educators. Nurse Education Today 24, 84–90.

Little, M. and Milliken, P. (2007) Practicing what we preach: balancing teaching and clinical practice competencies. International Journal of Nursing Education Scholarship 4(1), 1–14.

Manley, K. and McCormack, B. (1997) Exploring Expert Practice. London: Royal College of Nursing.

Manley, K., Hardy, S., Titchen, A., Garbett, R. and McCormack, B. (2005) Research Reports: Changing Patients' Worlds Through Nursing Expertise: Exploring Nursing Practice Expertise Through Emancipator Action Research and Fourth Generation Evaluation. London: Royal College of Nursing.

McCormack, B., Dewar, B., Wright, J., Garbett, R., Harvey, G. and Ballantine, K. (2006) A Realist Synthesis of Evidence Relating to Practice Development. Edinburgh: NHS Education for Scotland and NHS Quality Improvement Scotland.

McCready, T. (2007) Portfolios and the assessment of competence in nursing: a literature review. International Journal of Nursing Studies 44, 143–51.

National Statistics (2000) Standard Occupational Classification. [Online] http://www.statistics. gov.uk (accessed 1 July 2007).

NHS Quality Improvement Scotland (2007) Practice Development. [Online] http://www. nhshealthquality.org/nhsqis/1977.140.263.html (accessed 1 November 2007).

Nicklin, P. and Kenworthy, N. (2000) Teaching and Assessing in Nursing Practice London: Bailliere Tindall.

Nursing and Midwifery Council (2008) Standards to Support Learning and Assessment in Practice: NMC Standards for Mentors, Practice Teachers and Teachers. London: NMC.

Nursing and Midwifery Council (2004) The Prep Handbook. London: NMC.

Quality Assurance Agency for Higher Education (2001) The Framework for Higher education Qualifications in England, Wales and Northern Ireland. [Online] http://www.qaa.ac.uk/ academicinfrastructure/FHEQ/EWNI/default.asp (accessed 1 November 2007).

Quinn, F. and Hughes, S. (2007) Quinn's Principles and Practice of Nurse Education, 5th edn. Cheltenham: Nelson Thornes.

Royal College of Nursing (2003) Defining Nursing. London: Royal College of Nursing.

Sale, D. (2005) Understanding Clinical Governance and Quality Assurance. Basingstoke: Palgrave Macmillan.

Scottish Credit and Qualifications Framework (2003) An Introduction to the Scottish Credit and Qualifications Framework, 2nd edn. Edinburgh: SCQF.

Stephenson, J. (1998) The concept of capability and its importance in higher education. In Stephenson, J. and Yorke. M. (eds), Capability and Quality in Higher Education. London: Kogan Page Ltd.

Styles, M. (2005) Regulation and profession building: a personal perspective. International Nursing Review 52, 81–2.

Unsworth, J. (2000) Practice development: a concept analysis. Journal of Nursing Management 8(6), 317–26.

Watson, D. (2000) Lifelong learning and professional higher education. In Bourner, T., Katz, T. and Watson, D. (eds), New Directions in Professional Higher Education. Buckingham: Open University Press.

Watts, C. (2000) Issues of professionalism in higher education. In Bourner, T., Katz, T. and Watson, D. (eds), New Directions in Professional Higher Education. Buckingham: Open University Press.

CHAPTER 14

The Higher Education Perspective

Marilyn Fitzpatrick

CHAPTER OBJECTIVES

Aim

To examine the partnership approach to student education and development provided by the academic tutor in the higher education institution and the Practice Teacher.

Learning outcomes

■ Explore the relationship between the HEI and the placement educator.

■ Examine how these complement each other in the supervision and assessment of students.

■ Analyse the Practice Teacher's contribution to curriculum development.

The relationship between the higher education institution and the Practice Teacher

Placement learning is highly valued by students (Burrill *et al.* 2006) as it provides a means of developing knowledge and skills of direct relevance to their actual or intended field of employment. Many students undertaking a nursing or allied health professions course spend up to 50 per cent of their time in practice

(Universities UK, 2003) and practitioners play a key role in helping students to develop practical skills and apply knowledge gained from their studies. However, practitioners' contributions to students' educational experiences are not limited to those provided in the work place; they expand into other areas such as course development, quality monitoring activities and higher education institute-based teaching. This chapter provides a higher education perspective on how practitioners can provide input to each of these areas and how higher education institutions can prepare and support them in their practice teaching role.

It is essential to ensure that health and social care courses are rooted in the reality of practice and that the needs of the service area are addressed. Courses are continually being devised or revised and many practitioners working at the patient/client interface will have experienced some involvement with course development. The level of consultation will vary according to the nature of the course but where placement experience is a significant feature, the involvement of practitioners with a specific responsibility for practice teaching is crucial. A course specification must clearly detail placement resources and the higher education institution's mechanisms for supporting students in the practice setting (The Quality Assurance Agency for Higher Education (QAA), 2001, 2003; (Health Professions Council (HPC), 2005; HLSP, 2006)).

=============================== **ACTIVITY 14.1** ===============================

Examine the course documentation that you are required to complete for a student studying in your setting. Does it provide adequate information about the assessment? Have you received sufficient training to complete this documentation? Did you contribute to the creation of this document?

Once admitted to a course, students will normally be exposed to a variety of learning experiences. The 'theory–practice' gap is well documented in the literature, particularly in relation to nursing (Henderson, 2002; Landers, 2000), and one of the main challenges in health care education is to present curriculum content in a way that is meaningful to students and promotes the application of knowledge in the practice setting. Shardlow and Doel (1996) writing about social work education advocate practice-led curriculum, stating that the practical experience should precede the theoretical knowledge in order to enable students to then be able to more easily relate the theory to the relevant practice. Such a scenario has obvious benefits and may be feasible in social work education which stipulates that students must complete, as a minimum, 1200 hours placement experience in two practice settings and with two user groups (Department of Health, 2002). However, the practicalities of structuring a curriculum to allow placement experience to consistently precede higher education institution-based teaching poses particular challenges when statutory requirements for the practice component of a course are more demanding. For example, the European Directives for pre-registration adult nursing require students to gain experience with a wide variety of client groups and dictate that a total of 2300 practice hours must be completed in seven specified areas of practice (Nursing and Midwifery Council, 2004). Many of these areas are highly specialised and, due to limited placement capacity, it is unlikely that all students will be provided with similar experiences at the same point in time. Higher education institutions will endeavour to align theory input with practice experience but responsibility for teaching-related theory rests also with those accountable for facilitating learning in the practice setting.

One way of helping students to integrate theory and practice outside the practice arena is to involve practitioners in the delivery of the curriculum. Expert practitioners can take an active role by, for example, providing formal contributions to class room teaching. Such staff may be utilised to provide sessions on specialist areas of practice or to demonstrate how local practice innovations have been developed in response to the Government's health and social care agenda. They also may advise on how curriculum content may be presented in a way that is meaningful and relevant to the work setting.

=============================== **ACTIVITY 14.2** ===============================

What contribution have you made to the academic aspects of the student's learning? Do you visit the higher education institution? Can you easily communicate with their tutor? Do you feel that you have a good rapport with the tutors?

Work-based learning is also promoted as a way of reducing the 'theory–practice gap' (Swallow and Coates, 2004). Learning is grounded in the practice context and learning outcomes, related to and derived from the student's work role, are achieved through a planned programme of learning opportunities (Clarke and Copeland, 2003). There are various types of accredited work-based learning courses although all will comprise academic and practice components. Work-based learning is gaining popularity and the Department of Health (2004) advocates its expansion. However, its success depends on a collaborative partnership between the higher education institution and the organisation, and the latter's commitment to fostering a work culture that supports learning (Spouse, 2001).

The preparation of the Practice Teacher to perform their role

Whether students are undertaking a work-based learning course or one that has a placement learning component, the preparation of those who support learning in practice is an essential consideration for higher education institutions. Where a Professional Statutory Regulatory Body (PSRB) requires students to be allocated an appropriately qualified practitioner to support learning and assessment in the work setting, it is necessary to provide information on how such individuals will be prepared and supported in their role (HLSP, 2006; HPC, 2005).

=============================== **ACTIVITY 14.3** ===============================

What credentials or qualifications do you have as a Practice Teacher? How often do you refresh or update yourself?

Various labels are used to describe practitioners with a specific responsibility for supporting and assessing practice learning. Examples include, 'clinical educator' (Chartered Society for Physiotherapy, 2004; Royal College of Speech and Language Therapists, 2006), 'practice placement educator' (College of Occupational Therapists, 2006), 'mentor' and 'Practice Teacher' (NMC, 2008) and 'practice educator' (The College of Radiographers, 2006). Whilst the terminology may vary, a consensus exists that the quality of a student's placement learning experience pivots on highly motivated and appropriately prepared practitioners. The preparation of practitioners is as diverse as the titles used to describe their practice teaching roles. Not all health professions require their members to have a practice teaching qualification although most encourage participation in accreditation schemes that recognise practitioners' contributions to the education of the workforce. For example, the College of Occupational Therapists and the College of Radiographers have programmes based on the Accreditation of Clinical Educators (ACE) scheme developed by the Chartered Society of Physiotherapy (College of Occupational Therapists, 2006). Each incorporates six learning outcomes which differ only in the terminology used to describe their members and the context in which care is provided.

The Health Professions Council, which currently regulates 13 allied health professions, normally expects registrants who have a key role in facilitating practice-based learning to have undertaken 'appropriate practice placement educator training' (HPC, 2005, p. 7) but does not specify the nature of this preparation. The Nursing and Midwifery Council is more stringent in its requirements and adopts a staged approach to the mandatory preparation of practitioners who support learning and assessment in practice. The Nursing and Midwifery Council (2008) developmental framework incorporates four stages of preparation (not to be confused with academic levels of attainment), each with a specific set of learning outcomes classified under eight domain descriptors. The stages of preparation are independent and registrants may step on or off at any point along a continuum ranging from registrant (stage one) to teacher (stage four). The framework is somewhat complex as the minimum standards to be achieved differ according to the category of student that the practitioner will be working with. Pre-registration nursing students must be supported by a practitioner who has met stage two mentor or sign-off mentor standards, pre-registration midwifery students and post-qualifying students undertaking specialist practice or advanced nursing practice courses must be assigned a sign-off mentor, and students undertaking a specialist community public health nursing course must be supported and assessed by a Practice Teacher who demonstrates achievement of stage three outcomes.

In common with the accreditation schemes cited above, the Nursing and Midwifery Council framework offers experienced practitioners the option of demonstrating their achievement of the required standards in one of two ways, the programme route and the experiential route. Both will involve some form of assessment by a higher education institution (Chartered Society of Physiotherapists, 2004; College of Occupational Therapists, 2006; College of Radiographers, 2006; Nursing and Midwifery Council, 2008) although this may not be associated with the award of academic credits. Regardless of whether or not a practitioner has a recognised practice teaching qualification, they have a duty to ensure that their skills and knowledge are up to date and that they understand the requirements of the course that their student is undertaking.

================================ **ACTIVITY 14.4** ================================

Re-visit Chapter 2 and think about your responsibilities with regard to the requirements of your professional body.

A robust partnership between higher education institutions and placement providers is essential as the roles of lecturers, students, and those who support and assess practice learning need to be defined and agreed (QAA, 2001). Higher education institutions have a responsibility to ensure that practitioners receive sufficient information about a course and its expected learning outcomes in order to carry out their role. It is particularly important that assessment requirements are made clear and practitioners' fully understand how to apply marking criteria. The marking of practice learning is commonly on a 'pass' or 'refer' basis although the use of criteria to classify practice is established in some higher education institutions.

Assessing the student's practice

Classifying practice involves awarding a grade that distinguishes performance above (or below) that of the minimum standard required for a 'pass' but has been met with some scepticism in the United Kingdom. Calman *et al.* (2002) surveyed all Scottish institutions providing pre-registration nurse education programmes and found that only one had a system for grading clinical competence. Furthermore, this had been discontinued due to concerns about the subjective bias of practice assessors that had led to a number of high grades which were not in line with expected outcomes; factors which Canham (2001) and Walsh and Seldomridge (2005) have also noted as potential problems when using a practice classification system.

Canham (2001) reports on an exploratory study which preceded the introduction of an assessment system aimed at classifying the practice achievements of students undertaking a Community Specialist Practitioner programme. The assessment system was a product of collaborative work between existing practice educators, English National Board officers and the Course team and was first introduced in 1999 (alongside the existing assessment system as it was not until the following year that the practice component of the course would be treated as a level three, twenty credit unit).

Evaluation of the introduction of the new system revealed that the vast majority of practice educators awarded grades in excess of 70 per cent and Canham comments that, '...some practice educators may award marks for effort, despite contradictory written comments...' (p. 487) (the students' self-assessment marks formed a more normal pattern of distribution, suggesting that the marking tool was reasonably reliable). The findings raised a number of challenges but the assessment strategy was implemented the following year due to the enthusiasm of the practice educators and students, the course team's commitment to valuing practice, and the potential of the assessment tool. Subsequently, intensive work was undertaken by the course team and practice staff in response to the findings of the exploratory study and the evaluations. The method of classifying practice became firmly established and ongoing analysis of summative practice marks showed a more normal distribution (the majority fell within the bands 50–59 per cent and 60–69 per cent) indicating that positive outcomes can be achieved through a sustained commitment to joint ventures of interest to both higher education institutions and those who support learning in the practice setting.

The classification of practice remains a contentious issue for some higher education institutions and debates regarding its value mainly focus on concerns about the reliability of the assessment tool, the validity of outcomes, and subjectivity and consistency in relation to the assessment process (Andre, 2000; Williams and Bateman, 2003). These issues, however, are not confined to the use of classification systems: there is much evidence that they are equally problematic when assessment is based on a 'pass/refer' system (Andre, 2000; Chambers, 1998). Equally Practice Teachers may be ambivalent about 'grading' practice if they see this as being beyond their remit.

The Practice Teacher's contribution to assessment

Regardless of the system used to assess and record practice, higher education institutions are responsible for maintaining academic standards. This can be achieved by ensuring that practitioners with a specific responsibility for facilitating and assessing student learning have a clear understanding of the specified placement learning outcomes and the nature and process of the practice assessment. Such information may be conveyed, for example, through briefing sessions that take place in the university and during lecturers' visits to practice. Although these activities may be designed to inform practice staff of students' learning requirements and promote an understanding of the nature of any required assessments, they provide valuable opportunities for alerting university staff to practice issues that may be of particular relevance to the content and delivery of a course. These sessions can also provide a forum for higher education institutions and service staff to share their experiences, disseminate good practice, and provide peer support to colleagues. The latter may be particularly appreciated by those new to the practice teaching role; especially if they have not undertaken formal preparation.

ACTIVITY 14.5

Reflect on the ways have you been required to assess the student's performance? Do you feel that you could be objective and fair? What guidance did you receive regarding grading of work? Were you able to discuss this with academic tutors? Did you receive feedback on how your mark was moderated?

Practitioners who have successfully completed a higher education institution practice teaching programme will normally have their 'qualification' recorded in some way. The Nursing and Midwifery Council requires placement providers to maintain up-to-date registers of mentors and Practice Teachers. Employers are also responsible for undertaking triennial reviews to determine that their mentors and Practice Teachers can demonstrate the ability to meet Nursing and Midwifery Council criteria for remaining active on the local register (NMC, 2008). This system of quality monitoring is similar to that used in the ACE and APPLE schemes where accredited status is valid for five years at which point the onus is on the practitioner to provide evidence that they continue to meet the required standards (Chartered Society of Physiotherapists, 2004; College of Occupational Therapists, 2006).

The above systems are devised to ensure that practitioners meet the required standards laid down by their professional body. However, practitioners who support learning in the work place need not only to evaluate their own strengths and limitations but those of the placement organisation (Congdon *et al.* 2006) which must be conducive to learning. Evaluations must also be undertaken by higher education institutions as they are accountable for establishing and monitoring the quality of placements to ensure that students are provided with sufficient learning opportunities to achieve their learning outcomes (HPC, 2005; HLSP, 2006; QAA, 2001). Placement monitoring is normally undertaken via audits (Swann, 2002) which focus on factors such as the practice learning environment, student support mechanisms, the qualifications and experience of practitioners who support and assess learning, and strategies to protect the safety of both students and clients. The Practice Teacher is pivotal to establishing the learning culture within the organisation bringing education to field level. They are tasked with ensuring that relevant human and material resources are available to support the student.

Monitoring placement opportunities

To supplement audit data, information obtained from students' placement evaluations can provide a useful means of identifying examples of good practice as well as issues that may need to be addressed. Obtaining the views of practitioners who facilitate learning in the workplace is equally important as they are central to the success of placements. Higher education institutions need to be aware of any concerns in order for them to take remedial action such as providing additional support in the practice setting or developing better communication systems. Regardless of the nature and context of evaluations, action plans are required as a response to identified areas of general concern. Issues arising from these are normally fed into the higher education institution's quality monitoring systems and used in external audit processes.

ACTIVITY 14.6

In what way have you been required to assess the student's performance? Do you feel that you could be objective and fair? What guidance did you receive regarding grading of work? Were you able to discuss this with academic tutors? Did you receive feedback on how your mark was moderated?

External examiners have a crucial role in monitoring the quality of courses across organisations for parity. They are interested in the conduct of assessments and the strategies employed to ensure that students are treated fairly (Jinks and Morrison, 1997). One of the key functions of an external examiner is to make judgements about the rigor of assessment processes (QAA, 2004) and this applies to those used in both the higher education institution and placement setting. A sample of documentation submitted by students to support their achievement of placement learning outcomes will be seen by the external examiner. Many, but not all, students are required to submit a portfolio of learning to demonstrate their achievement of placement learning outcomes. Examination of students' work can provide external examiners with an insight into students' learning experiences and practice accomplishments.

It is considered to be good practice for external examiners to meet with students and their practice assessors. External examiners may wish to visit the practice area although, as Armitage and Karagic (2003) point out, such involvement is rare due to constraints on time and travelling. Therefore, meetings are most likely to take place on higher education institution premises. External examiners will normally meet separately with each party to encourage open discussion of practice learning and assessment experiences and to ascertain perceptions regarding the quality of information and support provided by the higher education institution. Occasionally, an external examiner may wish to meet with individual students and their assessors to verify the evidence and practice marking process but this is unlikely if the higher education institution can show evidence of a robust marking and internal moderation system.

The higher education institution perspective on education is multi-faceted and this chapter has covered only a few of the inherent issues. Higher education institution engagement with the service area has been advocated throughout as the main means of ensuring that contemporary health and social care education meets the requirements of both students and their employers. Students, service managers and practitioners who support learning in the practice setting have an unequivocal role to play in influencing both the design and the delivery of a course.

Curriculum design and delivery is increasingly focussed on the learning achieved in practice with the theoretical perspectives providing the underpinning structure to a curriculum that is driven by practice learning (Shardlow and Doel, 1996). More emphasis is being placed on key skills development and its assessment in the real-world situation. Practitioners are being encouraged to contribute to curriculum development and to teaching in the academic environment. This defines the crucial role of the experienced practitioner in educating the prospective workforce. Cultivating collaborative partnerships between higher education institutions and the service area is essential if the Government's vision of a highly skilled and educated professional workforce is to be achieved. It is essential that a strong relationship persists between the academic and practice-based staff as neither can function effectively without the other.

References

Andre, K. (2000) Grading student clinical practice performance: the Australian perspective. *Nurse Education Today* 20, 672–9.

Armitage, H. and Karagic, L. (2003) 'In Name Only' quality in practice assessment – is there a place for the external examiner? *Nurse Education in Practice* 4, 1–2.

Burrill, J., Hussain, Z., Prescott, D. and Waywell, L. (2006) An Introduction To Practice Education. [Online] http://www.practicebasedlearning.org/resources/materials/intro.htm

Calman, L., Watson, R., Norman, I., Redfern, S. and Murrells, T. (2002) Assessing practice of student nurses: methods, preparation of assessors and student views. *Journal of Advanced Nursing* 38(5), 516–23.

Canham, J. (2001) The classification of specialist student practice: results of an exploratory study. *Nurse Education Today* 21, 487–95.

Chambers, M. (1998) Some issues in the assessment of clinical practice: a review of the literature. *Journal of Clinical Nursing* 7, 201–08.

Chartered Society of Physiotherapists (2004) *Accreditation of Clinical Educators Scheme Guidance.* [Online] http://www.csp.org.uk/uploads/documents/csp_ace_scheme_guidance.pdf

Clarke, D. and Copeland, L. (2003) Developing nursing practice through work-based learning. *Nurse Education in Practice* 3, 236–44.

College of Occupational Therapists (2006) Guidance on Accreditation of Practice Placement Educators' Scheme (APPLE). [Online] http://www.cot.org.uk/public/education/accreditation/pdf/apple_guidance.pdf

Congdon, G., Wakins, G., Baker, T., Stewart, H., Thompson, E., Keenan, C. and Gibson, J. (2006) Managing the Placement Learning Environment. [Online] http://www.practicebasedlearning. org/resources/materials/intro.htm

Department of Health (2004) *Learning for delivery. Making connections between post qualification learning/continuing professional development and service planning.* London: DH.

Department of Health (2002) *Requirements for Social Work Training.* London. DH.

Health Professions Council (2005) *Standards of Education and Training Guidance.* London: HPC.

Henderson, S. (2002) Factors Impacting on Nurses' Transference of Theoretical Knowledge of Holistic Care into Clinical Practice. *Nurse Education in Practice* 2, 244–50.

HLSP (2006) Reviewer Handbook. [Online] http://www.hlsp.org/files/page/116720/HLSP_Reviewer_Handbook_v5.pdf

Jinks, A. and Morrison, P. (1997) The role of the external examiner in the assessment of clinical practice. *Nurse Education Today* 17, 408–12.

Landers, M. (2000) The theory-practice gap in nursing: the role of the nurse teacher. *Journal of Advanced Nursing* 32(6), 1500–56.

Nursing and Midwifery Council (2004) *Standards of Proficiency for Pre-registration Nursing Education.* London: NMC.

Nursing and Midwifery Council (2006) *Standards to Support Learning and Assessment in Practice. NMC Standards for Mentors, Practice Teachers and Teachers.* London: NMC.

Royal College of Speech and Language Therapists (2006) *National Standards for Practice Based Learning.* London: RCSLT.

Shardlow, S. and Doel, M. (1996) *Practice Learning and Teaching.* Basingstoke: MacMillan Press.

Spouse, J. (2001) Work-based learning in health care environments. *Nurse Education in Practice* 1, 12–18.

Swallow, V. and Coates, M. (2004) Flexible education for new nursing roles: reflections on two approaches. *Nurse Education in Practice* 4, 53–9.

Swann, B. (2002) An effective placement: creating a learning environment. Chapter 6. In: Welsh, I. and Swann, C. (eds), *Partners in Learning: A Guide to Support and Assessment in Nurse Education*. Oxon: Radcliffe Medical Press Ltd.

The College of Radiographers (2006) Practice Educator Accreditation Scheme. [Online] http://www.sor.org/public/practice-educator/pdf/practice-educator.pdf

The Quality Assurance Agency for Higher Education (2004) *Code of Practice for the Assurance of Academic Quality and Standards in Higher Education. Section 4: External Examining*, 2nd edn. Gloucester: QAA.

The Quality Assurance Agency for Higher Education (2001) Code of Practice for the Assurance of Academic Quality and Standards in Higher Education. Section 9: Placement learning. [Online] http://www.qaa.ac.uk/academicinfrastructure/codeOfPractice/section9/default.asp

The Quality Assurance Agency for Higher Education (2003) *Handbook for Major Review of Healthcare Programmes*. Gloucester: QAA.

Universities UK (2003) *Partners in Care: Universities and the NHS*. London: Universities UK.

Walsh, C. and Seldomridge, L. (2005) Clinical grades: upward bound. *Journal of Nursing Education*. 44(4), 162–8.

Williams, M. and Bateman, A. (2003) *Graded Assessment in Vocational Education and Training. An Analysis of National Practice, Drivers and Areas for Policy Development*. [Online] http://www.ncver.edu.au/research/proj/nr0008.pdf

Perspectives from Practice

The Patient

Patricia Rogers

The following is a patient's story. Excerpts from Patricia's personal diary document her experience. It is important to consider the patient or client's perspective of their care. Too frequently the voice of the patient is lost and they become overwhelmed by medical terms and well-intentioned professionals. In social work education the user's view is taken very seriously with service user involvement being a core aspect of programmes and user evaluation a mandatory part of student assessment. Various activities could be used to illicit the users view. This narrative can be used as an educational tool in any arena as the focus of an enquiry-based learning scenario for example.

Cancer, nurses and me

Patricia Rogers

16 January 2006: Everything is well with my world – until late in the evening I discover a lump in my left breast, it is pulling on the nipple making it inverted.

17 January 2006: My appointment with the doctor. The doctor is quite concerned and advises that he will refer me to a specialist.

25 January 2006: This was the day of my first encounter with the hospital that was to become like a second home over the next 18 months. Following a mammogram, biopsy and ultra scan (all carried out the same day as the Consultant was also unhappy with the 'lump') I was introduced to my Care Nurse and left hospital that day with the unofficial knowledge that, in every likelihood, I had breast cancer. My world had now collapsed around me.

How did I feel on leaving hospital? I was sick to the stomach, speechless. My husband, Paul had been with me on every step of the day and whilst I cried he held it together. In the car on the way home I feel we were both too frightened to say out loud what we were thinking. When I realised we were looking at cancer I immediately forgot any medical advancements that had been made and mentally went straight from the word cancer to coffin, and the panic rises up inside as the next thought in mind is "but I have a five year old, my daughter is only five!" and my head reeled with all the things in her life that I may not now be part of, and what of my Paul, how would he cope?

27 January 2006: Paul's father died. There is so much sadness in our home right now.

30 January 2006: Formal diagnosis; I have Infiltrating Lobular Cancer. Recommendation; mastectomy with reconstruction. The Consultant and Care Nurse were faultless in their treatment of me. The consultant was clear and concise and his manner was excellent. The Care Nurse was encouraging, supportive, sympathetic, unemotional and absolutely professional.

28 February 2006: I am booked into the Redwood Hospital, Surrey. I am surprised to learn that I get my own room with en-suite, as an NHS patient this wasn't expected. All of the nursing staff were very friendly and always smiling. Kindness exuded from them. The Registrar arrived to mark me up for the op. Consideration is given to the scaring so that it will be hidden by my bra. He asks if I would mind if a couple of students coming in. I confirm that I have no objections and am surprised to learn that apparently a lot of people won't allow students to be in attendance. Two young ladies came in. You would think I would be used to baring my breasts by now, but no. I still feel embarrassed and cannot look at the Registrar or the students whilst being examined. By now the nipple has returned more or less to normal, so unless you knew what you were looking at it wouldn't be apparent. The students commented to this effect. My recollection is that they were very quiet and shy, and that most of the talking was by the Registrar. However, I am sure that practical experience of being able to see what they learn about must be beneficial.

The following days spent in hospital I remember as not being at all unpleasant, probably due to the drugs! When the dressing was being checked or changed the nurses covered the mirror that was in the room, I was very grateful for that, as I was not at all interested in seeing what had been done to me. At all times the nursing staff were cheerful, chatty and professional.

My next encounter was with the District Nurses, and again they showed me tremendous kindness, nothing was too much trouble. These attributes are so very important in my opinion to the patient. As a patient I already felt slightly embarrassed about the whole performance of allowing a 'stranger' to see the results of my operation, so it was very much appreciated that they were chatty and matter of fact about what they were doing.

Chemotherapy was next on the agenda. The team of nurses who administered the chemotherapy cocktail to me were so cheerful to all the patients, very professional, considerate, and took an interest in the wigs and issues raised by the treatment. They always appeared to have time to chat. On a personal level chemotherapy is a horrible, horrible treatment, but a means to an end. You go in feeling fine, and in my case I knew two hours after the "cocktail" I would feel awful and would continue to do so for a fortnight. In addition one is losing one's hair and gaining weight! So the kindness and understanding of the nursing staff in sharing ideas of combating the various side-effects from the drugs and passing on information regarding wigs, hats, bandanas etc is priceless.

Radiotherapy; here the nurses were very efficient, professional and approachable. However, the radiotherapy works a little like a conveyor belt, not a lot of time for pleasantries. At this stage of the treatment I found this absolutely fine, the volume of patients dictates a quick turnaround, but equally I never felt that I was being rushed and attention to the detail in carrying out the procedure was always done with great care.

My only criticism would be that there appears to be an assumption on behalf of the medical world that the lay-person has a certain amount of knowledge, in respect of the healing process of wounds and what they should or shouldn't look like and when the healing is taking too long. In my case, I had no previous experience of wounds and therefore very much put my trust in the nurses, although I had been given a leaflet on leaving hospital about what to look out for I still put my trust in the nurses and I didn't have the confidence to question them. Unfortunately in my case this resulted in a wound that I spotted as potentially being infected being allowed to progress for a number of weeks, because the nurse I mentioned it to disagreed. Information advising what is considered normal within 48 hours of an operation if one is sent home the same day would also be extremely valuable.

Key points that made my treatment easier:

- The awareness that I already felt uncomfortable and embarrassed

- Being spoken to like a grown up

- Having a laugh with the nurses

- Being sympathetically and patiently dealt with, without being patronised

Ambulance Service Clinical Practice

Paul Jefferies and Heather Knight

Education and clinical supervision – the contemporary experience

Paramedics have traditionally been expected to work within the framework of their own clinical knowledge, many employers have utilised clinical guidelines to make this easier. These have varied but are increasingly being brought in line with national standards. The Joint Royal Colleges Ambulance Liaison Committee (JRCALC), an assembly of professionals from the field of medicine, nursing and the ambulance community have produced these guidelines bi-annually since the year 2000. The group reviews its guidance based on the principles of evidence medicine and best practice. The use of guidelines acts as a benchmark for adherence to best practice.

In the mid-1990s a limited number of Universities started to offer Higher Education Diploma and First Degrees in Paramedical Medicine. The higher education route was considered controversial as customarily the Operations Division of Ambulance Service Trusts were used to a demand-led approach to training and education. 'In House' courses meant that any sudden demand for skilled staff would lead to the provision of courses and the 'fast-track' approach has continued to be favoured over higher education.

A multiplicity of external factors is influencing the need for a major transformation of the provision of Ambulance Service Education. Perhaps the most influential is the move from vocational-based courses to higher education. Suspension of the IHCD in 2008–2009 has provided the impetus for a more rapid transferral to higher education providers.

At the time of writing, dual pathways for the provision of education exist concomitantly, access to Foundation Degree Courses and Paramedic Science

Degree Courses at local Universities and in-service provision of IHCD Courses. The influence of higher education represents a departure from the customary absolutist formal learning advocated by the IHCD and encourages a transition towards independent and contextual knowledge recognising the merit of experiential learning within the clinical field. This represents a dichotomy for most ambulance services, with the need to recognise the enhanced value of clinical experiential learning and extended periods of education and balance this with meeting the demands of service provision.

Traditionally the role of mentor (Clinical Supervisor) attracted a higher band of pay scale and financial remuneration may have been the main motivator for the undertaking of the additional responsibility. Clearly this strategy may have had a detrimental effect on the learner's experience, mentorship not necessarily being provided by an individual with a particular interest in the development and support of others. The transition to higher education has naturally necessitated an extension to the mentor and preceptorship period and individual ambulance services will need to accommodate this change with adaptation of the existing standard clinical supervision roles.

There is an increasing focus on selecting individuals to fulfil the mentorship role and some services have been proactive in seconding individuals to clinical teaching, supervision and mentorship modules delivered at local universities and higher education centres. There is also an obligation to provide training to existing clinical supervisors to ensure that they have an appreciation of the rigours of higher education, given that they are required to provide support and guidance to individuals undertaking university-based courses. The role is changing from that of the primary provision of clinical skills assessment to a more complex appreciation of the importance of reflective practice and an understanding of evidence-based medicine and the significance of critical appraisal.

In addition, National directives and policy documents such as *The Changing Workforce Programme* (DH, 2002), *Taking Health Care to the Patient* (DH, 2005), Emergency Access (DH, 2006) and the implementation of Call Connect (DH, 2007) have also informed the need to change with the emphasis on non-conveyance of clients to more appropriate client-centred pathways. National ambulance service demand has been estimated as rising annually by 6–7 per cent per year coupled with approximately only 10 per cent of the cases as a result of a life-threatening emergency (DOH, 2004). Paramedics undertaking higher education have been able to access a wider variety of clinical placements and received mentorship and support from a disparate range of health care professionals, including Nurse Practitioners, General Practitioners and Senior Hospital Doctors. This shift into the wider health economy has undoubted educational and developmental benefits and has been well received. But this transformational change requires a shift in assumptions and philosophy for the entire organisation.

There is a considerable need for individual ambulance services to provide enhanced training to its clinical supervisors in order to ensure that they are able to provide an appropriate level of support and guidance to the personnel undertaking university-based courses. This must include an understanding of the basic principles of research, critical analysis, evidence-based medicine and the importance of continuous professional development through self-directed learning and reflective practice. The role of clinical mentor remains in an embryonic stage for many services and there is a huge obligation for services to standardise the role and develop appropriate avenues for training and development.

References

Department of Health (2002) *The Changing Workforce Programme*. [Online] www.doh.gov.uk (accessed 1 March 2007).

Department of Health (2005) *Taking Healthcare to the Patient: Transforming the NHS Ambulance Service*. [Online] www.doh.gov.uk (accessed 1 March 2007).

Department of Health (2006) *Emergency Access*. [Online] www.doh.gov.uk (accessed 1 March 2007).

Department of Health (2007) *Call Connect: Access to Ambulance Services*. [Online] www.doh.gov.uk (accessed 1 October 2007).

Practice Teaching in Anaesthesia and Intensive Care

Graham R Nimmo and Ben Shippey

Anaesthesia and Intensive Care Medicine share many common factors in terms of teaching, training and education. They both occur in an acute hospital setting and traditionally an apprenticeship model has been prevalent. However, a number of changes have occurred recently in both service delivery and in medical training in the practice context and these have necessitated a revision of educational priorities and processes.

A number of potentially de-stabilising factors have come into play.

The European Working Time Directive (1998) resulted in the inception of Modernising Medical Careers (www.mmc.nhs.uk) which culminated in the introduction of the Foundation Programme (Foundation Curriculum, 2005). The precept was to improve patient safety and junior doctor working conditions by limiting the weekly hours of work. This has resulted in a reduction in actual hands-on service delivery by doctors who are now working around a third of the weekly hours which previous generations did. In many instances 'on call' activities have been replaced by the introduction of full shift rotas with interruptions to experiential learning and in particular, the loss of learning continuity: the ability to follow patients through their full clinical course and to learn the 'natural history of diseases' (Taylor, 1908) has been fragmented or lost. This is particularly the case when weekday working time is lost due to weekend shifts and, particularly night shifts.

These changes have also led to a re-examination of traditional professional roles with the acceptance of the concept of 'clinical competencies' being popularised (Competency Based Training in Intensive Care Medicine in Europe). One of the consequences of this is that activities which were traditionally the remit of medical staff are now being performed by others, in particular Advanced Nurse Practitioners (ANP).

So, at the same time as doctors weekly working hours are reduced, training time is shortened (with new run-through programmes) and other individuals are gaining the experience which these doctors would have previously accrued. The effects on patient safety are difficult to predict but interruptions (Chisholm *et al.* 2001; Nimmo and Mitchell, 2007) to continuity of immediate and ongoing patient care need to be compensated for by improved communication and team working (Hawryluck *et al.* 2002; Reader *et al.* 2007) and handover (Junior Doctors Committee, British Medical Association 2004). Situation awareness in this regard is pivotal.

Domains of Clinical Learning

Quite understandably there has been a traditional concentration on the more technical aspects of medicine including,

■ History taking

■ Clinical examination

■ Practical procedures

There are probably a number of reasons for this not least the fact that these activities are important. They are relatively easy to define, they can be repeatedly and fairly easily observed, and because of this assessment of them is well developed. In contrast, there has been a tardiness in embracing training, teaching and education in the non-technical domains (Croskerry, 2003) and in particular the cognitive and affective areas. This is in the face of the accrued evidence which demonstrates that as clinicians we spend a majority of our time thinking, deciding, feeling as opposed to hands-on *doing* (Croskerry, 2005, 2007). It could be argued that these non-technical activities (sometimes called human factors) merge with professional issues and behaviours.

At this point it is appropriate to highlight the crucial importance of clinical decision-making (Croskerry, 2005). The decisions which we are involved in are disparate and a non-exhaustive list could be: making a diagnosis; assessing prognosis; who to admit or discharge; decisions around the end of life; treatment limitation, withholding or withdrawing treatment or support, whether to attempt cardio-pulmonary resuscitation.

Team working, prioritisation (Fletcher *et al.* 2002), interruptions management (Alvarez and Coiera, 2005) and clinical handover all fit into this schema as important learning objectives.

Training, teaching and educational approaches

Planned teaching and learning experiences

It is possible to direct our clinical learners to a variety of learning resources which can be accessed readily through e-learning (two exemplars being the Scottish Intensive Care Society online tutorials and the European Society of Intensive Care Medicine PACT programme). In most teaching programmes there are also face-to-face tutorials and workshops on subjects appropriate to specific learner's needs.

In elective Anaesthesia there is still the opportunity for planned practical training, theoretical teaching and focussed learning in the operating theatre on a day-to-day basis and in the Intensive Care Unit ward rounds can incorporate teaching on patient management and can focus on clinical decision-making in particular. Any possibilities for supervised practice should be identified and capitalised on.

'Unplanned' teaching and learning experiences

So much learning in the acute clinical specialities relies upon the teacher and the learner seizing opportunities as they arise and incorporating both the practice of reflection on clinical experience and reflection on personal involvement into the cycle of learning (Usher, 2002). Part of the art of education in this context is to allow the learner to appreciate that they are undergoing a valuable learning experience despite the lack of tutorial room, whiteboard or power-point presentation. Of course, there are occasional 'clinical epiphanies' which can result in lifelong clinical behavioural changes (Blaney, 2005; Hogan, 2005).

Clinical learners should also be encouraged to 'set up' experiential learning. Taking the example of talking with families/patients they should ensure that they participate and observe situations where experienced staff are talking with patients, family, friends and they should be encouraged to pick out things which work and spot things which don't in order to incorporate 'best practice' from their own observations into their own practice.

Extended supervision

In this way novice learners initially manage patients under immediate supervision and as they gain experience and competence this supervision becomes less immediate, for example, in the theatre or room next door. As competence increases and experience is gained the supervision can become less local, for example, in the hospital or from places off site. The concept underpinning this is that the ultimate educational objective is to produce consultants who can function and work independently in the realisation that they don't suddenly metamorphose overnight when they take up their consultant post.

Patient safety

This area deserves special mention. It has been proposed that a curriculum for the teaching of patient safety should be developed in the acute specialities such as Emergency Medicine (Cosby and Croskerry, 2003) and Intensive Care (Fox-Robichaud and Nimmo, 2007).

Summary

There are many different approaches and methodologies underpinning clinical training and education. These should be conceptualised as a *repertoire* which can be used to construct a customised teaching programme for individual learners and for individual units. The important elements are the production of achievable learning objectives and the harmonisation of planned and opportunistic learning experiences to allow these to be attained.

References

Alvarez G. and Coiera, G. (2005) Interruptive communication patterns in the intensive care unit ward round. *International Journal of Medical Informatics* 74(10), 791–6.

Blaney D. (2005) The learning experiences of general practice registrars in the South East of Scotland. EdD Thesis University of Stirling.

Chisholm C., Collison, E., Nelson, D. and Cordell, W. (2001) Emergency department workplace interruptions: are emergency physicians 'interrupt driven' and 'multi-tasking'? *Academic Emergency Medicine* 8(6), 686–8.

Competency Based Training in Intensive Care Medicine in Europe. [Online] http://www.cobatrice.org/ (accessed January 2008).

Cosby, K. and Croskerry, P. (2003) Patient safety: a curriculum for teaching patient safety in emergency medicine. *Academic Emergency Medicine* 10(1), 69–78.

Croskerry, P. (2003) Cognitive forcing strategies in clinical decision making. *Annals of Emergency Medicine* 41(1), 121–2.

Croskerry, P. (2005) The theory and practice of clinical decision making. *Canadian Journal of Anesthesia* 52(6), R1–R8.

Croskerry, P. (2007) Commentary: the affective imperative: coming to terms with our emotions. *Academic Emergency Medicine* 14, 184–6.

European Society of Intensive Care Medicine PACT Programme. [Online] http://www.esicm.org/Data/ModuleGestionDeContenu/PagesGenerees/03-education/0B-pact-programme/25.asp (accessed January 2008).

European Working Time Directive (1998). [Online] http://www.incomesdata.co.uk/information/worktimedirective.htm

Fletcher, G., McGeorge, P., Flin, R., Glavin, R. and Maran, N. (2002) The role of non-technical skills in anaesthesia: a review of current literature. *British Journal of Anaesthesia* 88, 418–29.

Foundation Curriculum: Curriculum for the foundation years in postgraduate education and training (2005). [Online] http://www.mmc.nhs.uk/download/FP_Curriculum.pdf

Fox-Robichaud, A.E. and Nimmo, G.R. (2007) Education and simulation techniques for improving reliability of care. *Current Opinion in Critical Care* 13(6), 737–41.

Hawryluck, L., Espin, S., Garwood, K., Evans, C. and Lingard, L. (2002) Pulling together and pulling apart: tides of tension in the ICU team. *Academic Medicine* 77(10), s73–s76.

Hogan, P. (2005) The politics of learning and the epiphanies of learning. In Carr, W. (ed.), *The Routledge Falmer Reader of Philosophy of Education* pp. 89–91. Abingdon and New York: Rouledge.

Junior Doctors Committee British Medical Association (2004) Safe Handover: Safe Patients. Guidance on Clinical Handovers for Clinicians and Managers. [Online] http://www.bma.org.uk/ap.nsf/content/handover

Modernising Medical Careers. [Online] http://www.mmc.nhs.uk/pages/home

Nimmo, G.R. and Mitchell, C.M. (2007) An audit of interruptions in intensive care: implications for safety and quality. *Intensive Care Med.* 33(Suppl 2), S198.

Scottish Intensive Care Society online tutorials. [Online] http://www.scottishintensivecare.org.uk/education/icm%20induction/index.htm (accessed January 2008).

Modernising Medical Careers. The Next Steps. The Future Shape of Foundation, Specialist and General Practice Training Programmes (2005). [Online] http://www.mmc.nhs.uk/pages/resources/keydocuments

Reader, T., Flin, R., Mearns, K., and Cuthbertson, B. (2007). Interdisciplinary communication in the intensive care unit. *British Journal of Anaesthesia*, 98, 347–52.

Taylor, F. (1908) *A Manual of the Practice of Medicine* p. 6. London: Churchill.

Usher, R. (2002) Textuality and Reflexivity. IN Scott D. and Usher R. (eds). *Understanding Educational Research*. London: Routledge.

Mental Health

William Jackson

Over the past twenty years the landscape of mental health nursing has changed beyond recognition. The first ten years of these twenty saw the vast majority of the Victorian asylums finally closed. This ensured a significant educational and learning change for all those involved in mental health services, in particular the move from institutional to community settings.

In the most recent ten years, mental health, along with the NHS as a whole has experienced profound changes with emphasis upon modernisation and service user-centred care (DoH, 2000). In mental health this has culminated in changes in service delivery (DoH, 1999), policy implementation (DoH, 2001a) and significant legal changes (DoH, 2007). At the very heart of these changes, there is a demand for staff to work more closely and learn from and in multi-professional settings, examining their roles, responsibilities and skills (DoH, 2001b, 2004, 2006; Sainsbury Centre for Mental Health, 2001). Indeed, the Chief Nursing Officer's review of Mental Health Nursing has compounded the need for the development of skills within mental health nursing (DoH, 2006a) and this has presented a key opportunity and role for practice teaching to fulfil many of the recommendations advocated.

Such changes have clearly brought practice teaching as an integral part of the learning process. For some (Neary, 2000; Quinn and Hughes, 2007) the learning process clearly falls into two distinctive areas these being education and training (with specific teaching for this). Education is explained as a learning process that requires a complex synthesis of principles, values, skills and knowledge to solve problems.

Training is seen as a learning process for repeating skills and sometimes uniform performances which can be integrated into quality standards and criteria to produce (usually) known outcomes. Training and clinical teaching involves opportunities for learners to be exposed to new clinical skills and enhance existing ones. Such opportunities in mental health settings can range from a systematic procedure, such as a depot injection to more complex skills such as assign an individual's mental state were many variables need consideration.

Learning from clinical settings also lends itself to three core concepts that have been considerably well embraced within mental health nursing. These being experiential learning, or learning by doing, competency-based learning and clinical supervision.

Experiential learning has been eloquently explained by Schon (1991) and Kolb (1984). In clinical mental health settings a great deal of learning can and does, take place this way and in particular through observation. Competency-based learning has been evident in mental health nursing (and other branches) for many years and is set to expand. The growing significance of widening participation into mental health nursing, utilises national vocational qualifications and the concept of lifelong learning, both of which are underpinned significantly, by competency-based learning (CSIP/NIMHE, 2006; DoH, 2006b). For good practice to prevail it is important that clinical teaching includes opportunities for learners to rehearse, present and reflect in varied and complex clinical situations. This brings us to the third core concept which is clinical supervision. The prevalence of clinical supervision in mental health nursing has become an essential arena for practice to be enriched, while at the same time enhancing quality, learning and professional accountability for ones practice.

In mental health settings there are a number of possible clinical teaching and facilitating methods including, lectures, small group discussions, computer/information technology-based teaching and learning, problem-based learning, case-based learning, clinical scenarios, and structured observation. In the context of this brief overview it would not be possible to discuss all the teaching methods identified above, however, structured observation will be highlighted briefly as a strategy. Barker (2004) and Dickens et al. (2006) suggest that observation is a key skill in mental health practice; however, its employment has not always been seen as a learning opportunity, but more of a custodial duty. When observations become structured they become an integral part of practice teaching in mental health settings. When learners use structured observations on service users they can go beyond risk and safety, and assist in the assessment and monitoring of mental state changes, enhance therapeutic engagement by encouraging the development of interest in a trusting and meaningful way, formulate individualised care and facilitate the recovery process. When learners adopt structured observations of other professionals they learn how decisions are made and arrived at, team and group dynamics, collaborative processes and the interaction and engagement skills of other professionals.

Observation is central to clinical teaching in mental health; little can be achieved without it. It can and should be structured, active and purposeful, which can address both competency-based skills and those that are more complex. By requesting learners to simply 'observe' or allocating someone 'observation duties' is not sufficient. There is also an underlying assumption made at the point of these requests that the learner knows comprehensively, what they are observing for and why. Also, very rarely if at all, is this taken further to reflection, to unpack questions of how and gain a deeper and more meaningful understanding. Structured observation would purposely involve who, what, how and when. If this is added to reflection then this becomes a very powerful mechanism that can be applied to any given situation.

The number of combinations for teaching and learning situations that can be added to structured observation and reflection are many. One particularly useful area which can be used with great frequency is using structured observation with the mental state assessment. Accurate assessment of an individual's mental state is crucial, and required constantly within mental health settings. If a learner is introduced to the mental state assessment then he integrates this into his structured observations, this then, takes on a detailed, meaningful gathering of evidence-based features. This could be enhanced further by offering learners a pocket-sized mental state assessment card which can be used as a point of reference.

Structured observation can also be utilised in many other varied aspects of mental health nursing such as multi-disciplinary team work, assessment and various interventions. Within the confines of this text, only one method has been highlighted and as already been alluded to, there are a number of others, all of which have their own individual merits.

References

Barker, P.J. (2004) *Assessment in Psychiatric and Mental Health Nursing: In Search of the Whole Person*. Kingston Upon Thames: Nelson Thornes.

Dickens, T. *et al.* (2006) Therapeutic engagement through observation. *Mental Health Practice* 9(5), 26–7.

Care Services Improvement Partnership / National Institute Mental Health England (CSIP/ NIMHE) (2006) *10 High Impact Changes in Health Care*. London: CSIP/NIMHE.

Department of Health (2007) *Mental Health Act 2007*. London: DH.

Department of Health (2006a) *From Values to Action: The Chief Nursing Officer's Review of Mental Health Nursing*. London: DH.

Department of Health (2006b) *Learning for a Change in Health Care*. London: DH.

Department of Health (2004) *The NHS Knowledge and Skills Framework (NHS KSF) and the Development of the Review Process*. London: DH.

Department of Health (2001a) *The Mental Health Policy Implementation Guide*. London: DH.

Department of Health (2001b) *Working To-gether – Learning To-gether. A Framework for Lifelong Learning for the NHS*. London: DH.

Department of Health (2000) *The NHS Plan: A Framework for Investment, A Plan for Reform*. London: DH.

Department of Health (1999) *The National Service Frameworks for Mental Health: Modern Standards and Service Models*. London: DH.

Kolb, D.A. (1984) *Experiential Learning*. New Jersey: Prentice Hall.

Neary, M. (2000) *Teaching, Assessing and Evaluation for Clinical Competence: A Practical Guide for Practitioners and Teachers*. Cheltenham: Nelson Thornes.

Quinn, F.M. and Hughes, S. (2007) *Quinn's Principles and Practice of Nurse Education*. Cheltenham: Nelson Thornes.

Schon, D.A. (1991) *The Reflective Practitioner: How Professionals Think in Action*. Adershot: Ashgate.

Sainsbury Centre for Mental Health (2001) *The Capable Practitioner*. Salisbury: SCMH.

Occupational Health Nursing

Rosemary Shaw

Occupational Health Nursing has seen various changes from an educational point of view in the last twenty years. Many influences have contributed to these changes in practice such as the standards of proficiency for specialist community public health nurses from the Nursing and Midwifery Council (2004) and various Department of Health and Scottish Executive health policies. These will be discussed considering the impact on Occupational Health Nursing practice.

Occupational Health Nursing has changed from requiring little formal qualification with more focus on vocational training to the establishment of university degree programmes and the setting of Nursing and Midwifery Council Standards of proficiency for specialist community public health nursing (NMC, 2004). Occupational Health nurses now appear on the third part of the Nursing and Midwifery Council register upon successful completion of a specialist public health degree or being migrated via a portfolio (NMC, 2008). Occupational Health is clearly part of the Public Health agenda with practitioners ranking alongside health visitors and school nurses as specialists in the public health field. With degree programmes focusing on public health this provides the student with an opportunity to experience a range of different settings and areas of practice which will enable students to develop an understanding of the breadth and depth of specialist community public health nursing practice.

Recent government strategies have increased the profile of Occupational Health. For example, Securing Health Together (Health and Safety Executive, 2000) is the Government's ten year occupational health strategy and was launched in July 2000. Derek Wanless reviewed his 2002 report – 'Securing Our Future Health' Taking a Long Term View – this focused on prevention. It is clear that the need for an Occupational Health service has become a necessity.

Occupational Health practice has therefore developed with higher level skills required to meet the needs of the ever-changing workforce and the types of organisations that Occupational Health Nurses are required to work in. This has changed from the typical nurse in a factory situation to a professional who has a post-registration qualification. Following this route, the Occupational Health Nurse would have completed three years pre-registration education followed by additional education up to degree level. Working at degree level would include reflection on and in practice, the use of critical thinking skills and enhanced decision-making skills. The philosophy of post-registration courses is for students to develop the skills of lifelong learning, developing as reflective practitioners with the ability to problem solve, make sound clinical judgements and adapt to new situations within Occupational Health Nursing practice.

Increasingly, organisations wish to employ an Occupational Health Nurse that has gained a Nursing and Midwifery Council approved qualification in Occupational Health or are working towards that qualification. This may partly be due to the enhanced profile of Occupational Health within a generally more 'risk aware' business culture. A more proactive philosophy has evolved thus enabling Occupational Health Professionals to play a valuable role in ensuring compliance with Health and Safety Legislation, managing sickness absence and promoting health within the workplace. However, looking at the Specialist Community Public Health Nursing standards (NMC, 2004), it seems we have a clear challenge as a profession. Many Occupational Health Nurses are being educated on a distance learning course which allows them to work in substantive posts gaining experiential knowledge. This has been described by Kolb (1984) as an effective way of learning and was one which suited Occupational Health and which helped to produce many experienced practitioners. The Nursing and Midwifery Council (2004) standards in relation to education will be challenging to implement within Occupational Hvealth. These standards (NMC, 2004) require students to be supernumerary, thus providing a conflict with the business reality of hiring someone who is capable of doing the job but who does not have a post-registration qualification. Higher education institutions when planning for future curriculum development will need to work closely with employers and other stakeholders to enable these standards (NMC, 2004) to be implemented. Some Higher education institutions already have elected to develop non-Nursing and Midwifery Council approved courses as the challenges are too difficult to overcome.

The reality is that many of those seeking a Specialist Public Health qualification do so whilst in employment and are therefore required to be supported by a Practice Teacher as the NMC standards stipulate. However, it is almost impossible to find an appropriately qualified Practice Teacher to perform this role as it is not a well-established role in this specialism. Existing Practice Teachers will need to address any transitional educational requirements to meet these standards, as migration by portfolio is the suggested option, whereas future Practice Teachers will need to undertake an NMC approved course (NMC, 2008). This must be considered within future curriculum development.

A central mechanism of support for Occupational Health Nurse students is that provided by a suitably qualified Practice Teacher. Traditionally,

Occupational Health Nurses supported each other. More recently a Practice Teacher if available provides this support. Some Occupational Health Nurse students have access to such a person in their own organisation while others work on their own and need to be supported by a Practice Teacher from another organisation. Occupational Health Nurses work in various settings from heavy engineering to the NHS and can be employed by an organisation or through an Occupational Health provider. This can cause many challenges for the student who is undertaking a degree course at a distance and has a Practice Teacher from another organisation. The challenges include finding the time to meet to discuss learning outcomes and practical opportunities with the Practice Teacher. In addition to this, conflicting loyalties between the respective organisations of student and teacher may prove problematic. Mainly due to budget constraints the Practice Teacher may find it difficult to accommodate and support the student to the fullest extent. The Nursing and Midwifery Council has acknowledged the challenges of implementing the Practice Teacher standards and Occupational Health Nurses have a reprieve until 2010 for implementation (NMC, 2007).

Looking forward, the use of online learning will enhance the opportunity for students to interact with each other and get the much-needed peer support, and Practice Teacher support, especially if the student is enrolled on a distance learning course. Opportunities for discussing practical experiences confidentially with other students will increase the students' understanding and critical thinking skills. Communication between student, lecturer and Practice Teacher can be developed using online methods and while this mode of delivery is still in its infancy further exciting developments are being made.

Having a recognised Practice Teacher to support the Occupational Health Nurse student will enhance and develop students working at degree level. Despite the challenges, if the higher education institutions work in collaboration with organisations and relevant stakeholders the issues could be resolved.

References

Health and Safety Executive (2000) *07/00 Securing Health Together.* London: HSE.

Kolb, D.A. (1984) *Experiential Learning.* New Jersey: Prentice Hall.

Nursing and Midwifery Council (2004) *Standards of Proficiency for Specialist Community Public Health Nurses.* London: NMC.

Nursing and Midwifery Council (2007) *Circular 08/2007 Deferment of Practice Standards.* London: NMC.

Nursing and Midwifery Council (2008) *Standards to Support Learning and Assessment in Practice.* London: NMC.

Wanless, D. (2002) *'Securing our future Health' Taking a Long-Term View.* London: DH.

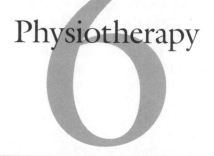

Physiotherapy

Rebecca Gilbert

The ultimate aim of undergraduate physiotherapy programmes is to create physiotherapists who not only have a good knowledge base but who also possess skills that enable clinical decision-making and practical competence. In order to gain these skills students have to complete at least 1000 hours of clinical practice as recommended by the Chartered Society of Physiotherapy (CSP), in different areas of physiotherapy, for example, neurology, respiratory and musculoskeletal. Practice placements vary from just a few days observation in the first year to up to six weeks by the third year. Each placement requires the same core skills such as communication but also encourages the development of skills specific to the individual area. Students will be expected to show an improvement in their knowledge and skills as the placements progress. By the third year students will be expected to carry their own caseload, work as part of a Multidisciplinary Team (MDT) and show well-developed clinical reasoning skills. Clinical placements must adhere to and educate the students on the 'Core Standards of Physiotherapy Practice' (CSP) (2005) and the 'Rules of Professional Conduct' (2002).

Students arrive on placement with different skills and experiences. It is therefore essential that both the student and the clinical educator are aware of their responsibilities and that it is explained to the student at the beginning of their placement what will be expected of them and how their learning will be assessed. It is the role of the clinical educator to treat each student individually and provide them with a wide range of learning experiences to improve their knowledge and to undertake appropriate assessment techniques to support this learning. This can only be done effectively if both the student and the clinical educator are familiar with the placement guidelines and assessment criteria set out by the CSP (2003) and the university, and have carried out the necessary preparation and planning.

If the clinical environment is not conducive to the students' learning then the assessment criteria will be difficult to achieve. As students are expected to work as part of a team, every member of the clinical team will contribute to the students' learning environment and therefore have the potential to impact on the students' learning. It is therefore necessary for the whole team to be involved in the students teaching and assessment (Savin-Baden and Howell Major, 2004). This contribution from the team can consist of supervision and feedback and may often involve other professions such as occupational therapy, nursing and medical staff. Students can also receive valuable feedback and support from one another; this is recognised by the CSP which now encourages clinical educators to supervise more than one student (CSP, 2002). The university provides each student with a tutor who visits them during the placement to offer support to both the clinical educator and the student.

The assessment of practice placements often provides the clinical educator with a challenge because of the diversity and complexity of the skills that require assessment, for example, team working, communication, clinical reasoning and practical skills. Whilst some of these skills such as communication are easier to assess, one of the most difficult areas for a clinical educator to understand and assess is that of clinical reasoning. Clinical reasoning relies largely on the integration of propositional, craft and personal knowledge all of which will vary with individual students. As experts in their field, clinical educators use forwards reasoning to solve clinical problems, often relying on previous experiences and craft knowledge to guide their thought processes. Students on the other hand use backwards reasoning, constantly testing hypotheses. It is important that clinical educators and students recognise the differences in their clinical reasoning and that the practice placement promotes practice that supports 'deep learning' in order to support the students' transition from novice to expert. Students need to be encouraged to test out hypotheses and draw on their previous experiences and form well-organised links between their knowledge and the clinical problems they face. In order to do this the student must be provided with a supportive environment, relevant experiences, and clinical problems provided in context with their learning and the clinical educators must allow the students to learn from both their positive and negative experiences.

The assessment criteria for practice placements is set out by the university and this is complemented by the students' individual learning development plan (LDP) which is completed by the student in conjunction with the clinical educator. This document highlights learning objectives specific to the student and the placement and runs alongside the assessment objectives set out by the university. In order to successfully evaluate students' learning and achieve objectives it is necessary to have provided the student with appropriate learning opportunities and carry out appropriate assessment techniques. The LDP helps to identify learning opportunities which can be varied and include anything from patient contact to spending time with other disciplines to delivering presentations.

In order to demonstrate the students' achievement a summative assessment must be carried out at the end of the placement (Cross *et al.* 2006). This assessment should follow the criteria set out by the university and have been monitored during the placement, often by the completion of a mid-way assessment. Assessment should also take place continuously throughout the placement providing the student with regular feedback. Only by regular assessment can a clinical educator identify the students' knowledge, clinical reasoning and progress, and therefore provide focus to the remainder of the placement and direct future learning. Regular assessment and feedback given constructively and using examples can have a positive effect on the student and shape their further motivation and development throughout the placement. By providing feedback and promoting reflection the clinical educator can encourage self-directed learning and evidence-based practice which are both equally important in lifelong learning and building the foundations of a career in physiotherapy. The assessment of practice placements when done effectively can be a positive experience for both the student and the clinical educator.

Resources

www.csp.org
www.practicebasedlearning.org

References

Cross, V., Moore, A., Morris, J., Caladine, L., Hilton, R. and Bristow, H. (2006) *The Practice Based-Educator. A Reflective Tool for CPD and Accreditation*. Chichester: John Wiley and Sons, Ltd.

Chartered Society of Physiotherapy (2005) *Core Standards of Physiotherapy Practice*. London: CSP.

Chartered Society of Physiotherapy (2002) *Rules of Professional Conduct*. London: CSP.

Chartered Society of Physiotherapy (2003) *Clinical Education Placement Guidelines*. London: CSP.

Chartered Society of Physiotherapy (2002) *Guidelines for Implementing Collaborative (Multiple) Models in Physiotherapy Practice*. London: CSP.

Savin-Baden, M. and Howell Major, C. (2004) *Foundations of Problem-Based Learning*. Berkshire: Open University Press.

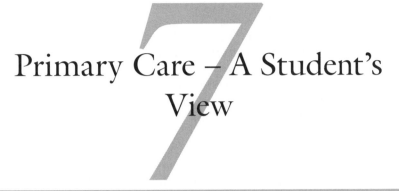

Primary Care – A Student's View

Alexis Halloran

Reflective Practice has been identified as key to professional development (Gibbs, 1988). Therefore, this narrative has given me the opportunity to critically analyse my own recent experience and what I ideally consider to be the role of a Practice Teacher. It was possibly the most daunting and emotional phase of my career to date. I worked alongside and was guided by a number of inspiring nurses and lecturers who together impacted greatly on my vision for the future as a District Nurse and I hope that I will be able to contribute to the journey of other students by offering my insights into the way a Practice Teacher can influence the progression of a student.

With the latest White Paper (Department of Health (DH), 2006) heralding a major shift in focus for care delivery within the community, it goes without saying that education will play a crucial role in preparing students for their future roles and responsibilities. Though any vocational course requires intensive study, this particular one can be greatly aided by a Practice Teacher's supervision technique and their ability to fulfil the roles of supporter and advisor in relation to both practical and theoretical skills.

The standard required of a Practice Teacher is very high as specific skills and knowledge are needed to support and develop the transition from Staff Nurse to District Nurse (Byers, 2002; Hudson, 2001; Nursing and Midwifery Council (NMC), 2001). A Practice Teacher needs to demonstrate the link between theory and practice and encourage the student to seek evidence to support their practice by looking at such theoretical perspectives as Carper's (1978) 4 Ways of Knowing and Sackett *et al.*'s (2000) definition of evidence-based nursing integrating the best research evidence with clinical expertise and patient values to improve patient outcomes. It de-emphasises ritual, isolated and unsystematic clinical experiences, ungrounded opinions and tradition as a basis for nursing practice stressing instead the use of research findings, quality improvement data, the consensus of recognised experts and the affirmed experience of substantive practice (DH, 1998; Sackett, 1996).

Their style of teaching should be tailored to each student's individual needs, as no two students are the same. At the beginning of the programme it is advisable for students to take an observational role; leading on to complete management under supervision towards the end. Students were often each others worst enemies when discussing their experiences, as they varied widely this often led to some questioning their capability and lengthy discussions on whether their various mentors had confidence in their ability. Therefore, it is important to discuss a student's learning needs and draw up an individual learning contract that supports their own professional development.

The introduction of nurse prescribing has emphasised their role as independent practitioners for many community nurses and promoted the idea that nurses, given appropriate training can be competent to diagnose, treat and deliver appropriate care to their patients (Winterburn and Lodge, 2004). This autonomy can be promoted, when it comes to first assessment visits as the Teacher could first let the student observe, then move on to observing the student and then to the student going solo. This again is a nurtured approach, beneficial to knowledge and confidence building. It can lead to professional development for both the student and the mentor, observing each other's practice and learning from it. Learning through reflection should also be encouraged, for instance if a mistake is made, allow this to happen (without putting patients at risk) and then discuss the positives and negatives, always making sure even if there are more negatives than positives, a positive is highlighted, avoiding knocking the student's confidence.

Following the observational stage, Practice Teacher's should advance the student by taking their own small caseload of patients encouraging them to take their time and keep a reflective diary, which will help them to develop and look at their practice, moving away from the concept of task working. This is something I think we tend to do when working as staff nurses. Kolb's (1984) experiential learning cycle highlights that for learning to occur the student must be provided with opportunities to allow them to build on their existing knowledge and experience and thus help them to develop new skills in holistic assessment and decision-making by looking at the patient as a whole. Training the student to constantly question their rationale for doing things is essential, that is, are there any guidelines or protocols promoting best practice. In addition, it can help them to prepare for first assessment visits, making the holistic approach their natural approach.

Eventually, the student should be encouraged to act up to team leader with the supervisor taking a complete step back. Keeping this towards the end of the placement allows the student to grow and develop into their new role and get the most out of their practice placement. Key words which define the ideal approach by the Practice Teacher are transitional but realistic, that is, not giving too much to start with but not being too easy going; developmental, a strong theory to practice approach, encouragement to reflect and consider all areas of specialist practice and an understanding of strong leadership.

A key element of leadership is using the talents and the skills of team members and the strengths they bring to the team. Many tools are available to help individuals diagnose their strengths such as the Myers Briggs Type Indicator (Briggs-Myers, 1995). This focuses on whether the individual is an extrovert or introvert and can help to indicate how they would work best and what would stimulate them to perform more effectively in the group.

Initially, students are extremely vulnerable, they are out of their comfort zone in a new team, and a new environment. Strategies that could be used to help the student settle into the team are supportive poems and team-building exercises to enable relationship building, encouraging and treating the student as a member of the team in a relaxed environment. These considerations help the student to function effectively in a supported learning context and as a consequence the student should feel less threatened or intimidated and will hopefully perform at a higher level.

References

Briggs-Myers, I. (1995) *Gifts Differing: Understanding Personality Type*. California: Davies-Black Publishing.

Byers, P. (2002) *Report on the Practice Educator Project*. London: Community Practitioners Health Visitors Association.

Carper, B. (1978) Fundamental Patterns of Knowing in Nursing. *Advances in Nursing Sciences*. 1(1),13–23.

Department of Health (1998) *A First Class Service: Quality in the New NHS*. London: HMSO.

Department of Health (2006) *Our Health, Our Care, Our Say: A new Direction for Community Services*. London: DH.

Gibbs, G. (1988) *Learning by Doing: A Guide to Teaching and Learning Methods*. Oxford: Oxford Polytechnic.

Hudson, R. (2001) *Practice Educators Preparing for New Roles in the New NHS*. London: Community Practitioners Health Visitors Association.

Kolb, D. (1984) *Experiential Learning*. Englewood Cliffs: Prentice Hall.

Nursing and Midwifery Council (2001) *Standards for Specialist Practice and Education*. London: NMC.

Sackett, D. (1996) 'Evidence-based medicine: what is it and what isn't it'. *British Medical Journal* 312(7023), 71–2.

Sackett, D., Strauss, S., Richardson, W., Rosenberg, W. and Haynes, R. (2000) *Evidence Based Medicine: How to Practice and Teach EBM*. New York: Churchill Livingstone.

Winterburn, S. and Lodge, E. (2004) Preparing nurses for 'first contact' in the management of minor illness. *Journal of Community Nursing* 18(9), 14–17.

Secondary Care

Abigail Cooper

Practice teaching within secondary care is undertaken in a dynamic and challenging environment. Clinical areas are increasingly busy, and there may be inadequate time for educators to ensure the placement is effectively teaching the practical skills required (Humphreys *et al.* 2000). Teaching is not always a formal process and learning takes place in a variety of contexts. For example, role modelling is a valuable method of displaying knowledge skills and attitudes for the learner to observe.

The introduction of the Nursing and Midwifery Council Standards (NMC, 2008) has introduced a new framework for nurse education and developed the structure for supporting learning in practice. This will have implications for mentors and Practice Teachers in terms of, for example, the introduction of the new 'sign off' mentor status. Mentors will need to demonstrate that they have competently 'signed off' three students in order to use the title of 'sign off' mentor. Practice Teachers have to mentor at least one student within a three-year period in order to maintain their Practice Teacher status. Implementing these processes will have an effect on a macro level as organisations will need to consider workforce planning to ensure they have adequate appropriately educated staff to fulfil the required roles.

In order to support the increasing numbers of students in practice different models have been adopted. More commonly a team approach may be used to facilitate learning where although the student has one named individual the team work collaboratively in order to facilitate a learning environment conducive to student progression and development. This approach can promote inter-professional learning involving students from various disciplines to enhance the educational experience (RCN, 2000).

Commonly, secondary care is a learning environment for pre-registration nurses who will require a mentor and a sign off mentor in order to fulfill the NMC requirements. In addition, post-registration nurses who are advancing their roles will, for example, in prescribing and advanced practice require suitably qualified educators to facilitate their development and assess their practice. This is a role that currently may be undertaken by medical staff in terms of assessing diagnostic and medical examination skills. However, it is envisaged that as the number of nurses practicing at this level increases they will go on to become Practice Teachers to support future nurses in advancing their practice. During this period of transition the use of a 'buddy system' can support nurses as they develop their role as Practice Teachers (McAskill, 2007). A buddy is a named nurse who can act as a role model and support and facilitate learning alongside the medical assessor.

There are exciting opportunities to develop nurse education in secondary care. Different models may be adopted although it is crucial that the patient is kept at the centre of the process. Nurses who wish to develop their career but remain in clinical practice now no longer have to move in to a managerial role or higher education. Opportunities exist clinically to work at a higher level as has been acknowledged in roles such as nurse consultant or educationally focussed roles in practice.

References

Humphreys, A., Gidman, J. and Andrews, M. (2000) The nature and purpose of the role of the nurse lecturer in practice settings. *Nurse Education Today* 20(4), 311–17

McAskill, H. (2007) *Non-Medical Prescribing in Scotland: A Project Report.* Edinburgh: NHS Education for Scotland.

Nursing and Midwifery Council (2008) *Standards to Support Learning and Assessment in Practice.* London: NMC.

Royal College of Nursing (2000) *Presidential Taskforce on Nursing Education.* London: RCN.

Speech and Language Therapy

Carol Fairfield

Pre-registration undergraduate or Post graduate Speech and Language Therapy students attend clinical placements as an integral part of their programme. This practice-based learning needs to promote the development of skills and competencies identified by the QAA benchmark standards and Health Professions Council (HPC) Standards of Proficiency for speech and language therapists. Further guidance as to the levels of competencies needed is found in the competencies framework for clinicians identified by the Royal College of Speech and Language Therapists. More recently the National Standards for Practice Based Learning (RCSLT, 2006) have been produced. These latter standards incorporate the generic standards mentioned above, but provide profession-specific guidelines and good practice for Speech and Language Therapy placement-based learning.

The placement educator is a Health Professions Council registered qualified speech and language therapist. The Practice Educator supports a student's development in three main areas as identified by the QAA benchmark standards: the application of theoretical knowledge to clinical practice; development of technical skills such as assessment and the relevant interpersonal and communication abilities to establish and maintain the therapeutic environment. The Practice Educator thus facilitates the student's development of professional craft knowledge, as described by McAllister and Lincoln (2004). In addition, the DOH (2001) identifies the need for practitioners to be able to continue life-long learning and as such the teaching strategies employed by Practice Educator need to support this.

The Practice Educator thus needs to adopt a number of teaching strategies such as structured observation and modelling/demonstrating. The primary strategy used is experiential learning. This is defined by Higgs and Jones (2000) and Higgs and Edwards (1999) as more than just active learning. It requires the student to reflect on their actions within the clinical learning environment. The Practice Educator guides the student through the development of reflecting 'on an action' to 'reflection in action' (Jenson and Saylor, 1994) via providing the learning opportunities for them to practice and reflect on their skills ever more independently. Feedback by the Practice Educator is an essential part of this process. He/she provides regular ongoing feedback on patient sessions, as well as written and verbal feedback via a clinical report at the end of a placement.

The main challenge for the Practice Educator in facilitating experiential learning is to map their placement learning opportunities to the learning outcomes identified by the higher educational institution. Practice Educators work in a variety of settings and some placement areas lend themselves more to particular learning outcomes than others. The Practice Educator working in a consultative role, who visits schools, assesses children and provides advice may be able to offer more direct hands-on experience in assessment than a Practice Educator working elsewhere. In their own placement environment the Practice Educator identifies situations and clients suitable for student learning. Issues of caseload demand, student independence and learning styles of both student and Practice Educator will all impact on this, including the Practice Educator perception of risk to the client (Morris, 1998), which can potentially reduce the Practice Educator's confidence in letting the student gain valuable hands-on experience.

It is expected that students will work with the clients from the beginning of their placements and not just carry out structured observations. The Practice Educator is thus expected to identify and break down clinical tasks such as, carrying out an assessment or giving advice to a parent/nurse/teacher, using their experience and knowledge of a student and their target learning outcomes. The confidence in these decisions is shaped by training at the higher education institution, and also supported by clinical placement handbooks as well as ongoing contact with tutors at the higher education institution. The use of web-based resources available to the Practice Educator on university web pages for placement activity ideas, or the use of e-mail to support student feedback have all supported placement and Practice Educator development. Peer support within the speech and language therapy service enables clinicians to share good practice whenever possible.

Students who do not achieve their learning outcomes or who may be in advance of the learning outcomes may be problematic for a Practice Educator particularly if they are novice clinical educators. Specific processes for the Practice Educator in this situation are described in the RCSLT placement standards, identifying a need to work in a tripartite relationship with the student and the higher education institution as soon as a problem is identified.

It is expected that there is a programme of training available at the local higher education institution to support the Practice Educator's development as a clinical educator. This will generally include introductory workshops prior to a Practice Educator providing a placement and then a graded programme of workshops/training to support their Continuing Professional Development as an educator. The initial training will address all aspects of a placement including administration, teaching strategies and the development of feedback and marking.

Traditionally, Speech and Language Therapy placements have comprised a one-to-one Practice Educator: student model for a number of reasons such as the working environment (small rooms/peripatetic work with lots of time in the car) as well as a perceived potential increase in workload. However, many more varied placements are now offered with benefits of these being demonstrated (e.g. Parker and Kersner, 1998). Individual Practice Educators may provide peer placements which can vary from 2–8 students. The premise behind these models is the differing learning opportunities they provide, both in terms of variety of clients seen as well as peer learning. For example, group placements have been used in communication groups with adults with aphasia. The Practice Educator benefits from facilitating larger groups and the students learn both from each other as well as seeing a more diverse client base. A disadvantage to the Practice Educator is the number of final reports to be written and the management of students with different learning styles, but this seems to be overridden by the advantages.

A pilot mixed year placement took place in 2006. Second year (finalist) MSc students were joined on a weekly placement by either second or third year BSc students. Prior to the placement, all were given definitions of their role and responsibilities and example activities to achieve this. For example, each student year group was expected to give feedback to the other, with the focus and agreed target behaviours of feedback and reflection being relevant to their current level of study. The Practice Educator's role varied in this placement model, as they had to facilitate learning across and within year groups. This model promoted more of a team or collegiate approach and personal report indicated that in some cases this gave the Practice Educator more time, rather than less, within the placement. Feedback following the placement indicated that both sets of students identified specific benefits from this model. These results supported the aim of the model of placement provision, which was to engender peer learning between groups at different stages of their programmes without greater demand on the Practice Educator.

Using varied placement models is essential in the Speech and Language Therapy profession, not just to ensure sufficient placements but to continue to promote effective placement learning and be flexible enough to embrace the changing models of Speech and Language Therapy provision within the NHS and Education sectors.

References

Department of Health (2001) *Framework for Lifelong Learning in the NHS*. London: DH.

Health Professions Council. Standards of Proficiency. [Online] http://www.hpc-uk.org/assets/documents/10000529Standards_of_Proficiency_SLTs.pdf (accessed May 2008).

Higgs, J. and Edwards, H. (1999) *Educating Beginning Practitioners*. Oxford: Butterworth Heinmann.

Higgs, J. and Jones, M. (eds) (2000) *Clinical Reasoning in the Health Professions*, 2nd edn. Oxford: Butterworth- Heinmann.

Jenson, G.M. and Saylor, C. (1994) Portfolios and professional development in the health professions. *Evaluation and the Health Professions* 17(3), 344–57.

McAllister, L. and Lincoln, M. (2004) *Clinical Education in Speech-Language Pathology.* London: Whurr.

Morris, C. (1998) The hidden determiner of student learning opportunity on clinical placement. *International Journal of Language and Communication Disorders* 33, 238–54 (supplement).

Parker, A. and Kersner, M. (1998) New approaches to learning on clinical placement. *International Journal of Language and Communication Disorders* 33, 255–69 (supplement).

Royal College of Speech and Language Therapists (2006) *National Standards for Practice Based Learning.* London: RCSLT.

The Quality Assurance Agency for Higher Education Benchmark Statements: Health Care Programmes. [Online] http://www.qaa.ac.uk/academicinfrastructure/benchmark/health/default.asp (accessed May 2008).

Facing the Future

Anne Smith, Heather McAskill, Kirsten Jack

This book has provided an opportunity for those engaged in practice education to reflect on their role and analyse their skills as teachers. Whilst the practice setting is a rapidly changing and turbulent environment requiring practitioners to be flexible and responsive in their approach, Practice Teachers are charged with moulding the future workforce through their educational role. The necessity to maintain currency in their own practice, to work from a sound evidence and research base is paramount and then their responsibility is to disseminate that knowledge and expertise to students. The ultimate goal is to ensure that students qualify fit to perform the current and emerging roles to meet the needs of the population in the twenty-first century.

The governments within the four UK countries have published a raft of documents recounting their vision such as Our Health, Our Care, Our Say (DH, 2006) and these clearly articulate their intention to provide services that tackle the dominant issues concerned with waiting lists, and other key targets that affect the patient's journey.

However, the greatest implications for the NHS lie in the demographics of the population and the prospect of older people living longer and making greater demands on finite resources. The need to work smarter and more efficiently to meet these demands are focussing the minds of those with the responsibility to maintain quality services.

The Department of Health and Nursing and Midwifery Council (DH, 2007) have recently consulted with the nursing profession on their vision for a whole new approach to their educational system that will be more appropriate in meeting the challenges ahead.

This cannot be divorced from the recent publication 'Modernising Nursing Careers' (DH, 2004) which sought to modernise the image of nursing and build a more flexible workforce to deliver the new agenda. It is only one part of a larger programme to modernise all health care careers. The educational requirements that will be integral to such a recommendation are huge. Practice Teachers will be at the forefront of the implementation and must therefore be prepared to become involved and proactive in the design and delivery of programmes.

The Knowledge and Skills Framework (DH, 2004) has been adopted to provide an objective national framework on which staff reviews can be based. This applies to all professional groups. A key component of this is to embrace lifelong learning and adequately resource it so that individuals can map their career progression and be supported to achieve their goals. The investment in staff education and development is a central tenet of this framework. It indicates a 'joined up' approach as it applies across the professions and may be the forerunner of a similar approach to education. Inter-professional education is strongly advocated as the preferred option wherever it can be implemented as it is recognised that professional groups are more informed and operate more effectively if they learn with each other.

Health care is changing beyond recognition. It is being confronted with new challenges and this is the key driver for an educated workforce that has the ability to respond. The Practice Teachers' role is a lynchpin in supporting education and the development of practice so that the workforce is equipped to face the future.

References

DH (2007) *Towards a Framework for Post-Registration Nursing Careers: A National Consultation.* London. DH.
DH (2006) *Modernising Nursing Careers Setting The Direction.* London: DH.
DH (2004) *NHS KSF and the Development Review Process.* London: DH.

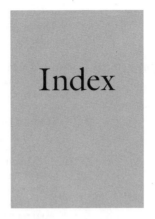

Index